Social Facilitation *in Action*

A Behavioral Intervention Therapy
for Individuals with Autism, Asperger's Syndrome,
and Other Related Syndromes

by Illana Katz *and* Andrew Yellen, Ph.D.

Published by
Yellen & Associates Psychological & Educational Services
Northridge, California
and
Real Life Storybooks
West Hills, California

Other works by the authors:
by Illana Katz–*Joey and Sam* (co-authored by Dr. Edward Ritvo); *Show Me Where It Hurts* (co-authored by Dr. Alan Rosenthal); *Uncle Jimmy; Sarah*; and *Hungry Mind-Hungry Body*.

by Andrew G. Yellen, Ph.D.– *Understanding the Learning Disabled Athlete* (co-authored by Heidi Yellen); and *The Art of Perfect Parenting and Other Absurd Ideas*.

FIRST EDITION Spring 2000

Proofreading Catherine Weinstein
Distribution David Katz
Cover Illustration Tyler West

Library of Congress Cataloging in Publication Data

Katz, Illana and Yellen Ph.D., Andrew G.
Social facilitation in action : a behavioral intervention therapy for individuals with autism, Asperger's syndrome and other related syndromes / Illana Katz and Andrew G. Yellen, Ph.D.
ISBN : 1-882388-15-1 : $39.95
1. autism (manual) I. Title

Printed in the United States of America

This book is dedicated to Seth
for all that he has taught us;
to the many unique and special people–big and little,
for all they have shown us;
and to the parents, educators and other professionals
for all they have shared with us.
Pen in hand we can make a difference.
And hand in hand we can change the world.

Table of Contents

Authors' Note

The terms "he," "his," "him" and "himself" should be understood to be interchangeable with their feminine forms. Likewise, in almost all cases where "child" or "children" is used, the reader should feel free to substitute "adult" or "adults." The concepts presented in this book are not gender or age specific. It is only for the sake of brevity and readability that the terms used were chosen.

Foreword

In 1996 Yellen & Associates, a psychological and educational services provider, was asked to be part of "Professionals Serving Autism." It was a group of professionals from different disciplines, including medicine, psychology, speech therapy, occupational therapy, physical therapy, and behavioral therapy. The group would meet once a month to share all the new information on autism. Dr. Ricki Robinson, herself the mother of a child with autism, was the founding force behind the group. We would try to have a presenter each time we met. So many new ideas and theories were coming up so rapidly it was important we all remained abreast of any advances.

Enter Illana Katz. A world-renowned author and also the mother of a child with autism, Illana knew she could successfully impact behaviors by writing out scripts. She promptly displayed several stories she had written for her son, Seth. She did not know exactly how to integrate the process into the mainstream of information available to other parents, but she knew she had to find a way. The results of her efforts were far too successful and important not to share with others.

I approached her after her presentation and asked her to meet me in our office the following morning. Illana became an integral part of Yellen & Associates' approach to serving the autism community. We first needed to have a name and title for what she did. Social Facilitation and Social Facilitation Consultant were born. The object all along has been to empower those working with individuals with autism. *Social Facilitation in Action* not only provides parents with a wonderful tool, but provides therapists with a whole new "lesson plan" of therapy and behavioral modification.

Though she will be embarrassed, let the world of autism know Illana Katz is a remarkable, compassionate human being who has given a gift to parents and therapists, alike. And we would like to share her efforts with you.

Andrew G. Yellen, Ph.D.

"Tell your readers something about your life, something which relates to this manual," Dr. Yellen said to me.

"Why?" I asked him.

"Because your readers need to know how close you are to this material," he replied. "Because you are a researcher, a writer and the parent of a child with a disability. Because you've been there."

Perhaps the good doctor is right. Perhaps you and I have a great deal in common. And perhaps knowing a bit about who I am will help us work through this manual together.

My life has been filled with opportunities and pitfalls, big ones and little ones. This manual is one such opportunity; an opportunity to help you, guide you, give you a tool, a method to help you help others.

I came upon this tool many years ago. It was long after the birth of our last son. His name is Seth and he is now a teenager. The youngest of four children, he would become the family's focus, in more ways than one.

As an infant, our new son had all the required parts and yet there was something more. Something just wasn't quite right. How many of you sensed something early on with your child, your loved one? For us, there was just this tiny bit of uncertainty surrounding our youngest.

What seemed different? His interest in the world seemed limited. Rattles kept slipping out of his grasp. There wasn't much interest in objects, no matter how colorful or mobile, whether they were close by or floating above his crib. At eight months of age we would find Seth rocking on his hands and knees in his sleep, or banging his head on the mattress of his crib. At a year he could spin coasters like a pro, but had almost no words. He didn't even wave bye-bye. At two years old he still wasn't pointing at things and used only about a dozen words, a dozen words mixed with baby babble.

Einstein didn't speak on time either, I assured myself. Nevertheless, in the pit of my stomach there was a sense of urgency, a sense that time was moving forward, yet our son was not.

Seth seemed like a happy baby, I reassured myself. He wasn't stiff. He would snuggle against us. He seemed to be affectionate. He had eye contact. He slept all night. Yet our uncertainty, our unnamed fears persisted until at age two and a half years old we could no longer avoid the obvious. This child was just not developing as his sister and brothers had. To the contrary, he appeared to be losing developmental ground. He seemed to almost disappear inside himself, losing some of the few words he had painstakingly developed, becoming far more silent and even abandoning the baby gibberish he had used so ubiquitously. He was becoming more and more distant, even appearing to be hard of hearing. It appeared he was withdrawing to a place we seemed unable to reach. Clearly our son had some kind of problem, some kind of serious problem.

Thus began our search for answers. In 1988 "high-functioning autism" as a sub-category of autism was not necessarily available in library literature. What did appear was information regarding autism in its more severe form. Having previously been fascinated by films and literature surrounding this strange syndrome it was not difficult to imagine that we were looking at some form of it when we observed the behaviors of our young son. Some of the symptoms discussed resembled those of our son, some didn't. And though there appeared to be significant differences, there were also significant similarities.

After many trips to countless doctors it would be Dr. B.J. Freeman who would pin the label on him. "Your son has autism," she said. "He seems to be high functioning; nonetheless, it is autism."

Thus began the challenge of a lifetime; how to take a child with a potentially devastating disability and help him find a life worth living, a life with meaning; how to protect him from a savvy world, a world from which he might always need to be protected.

That challenge led me to delve into the life of Albert Einstein, whose life and idiosyncrasies had always been of interest. Did Einstein have some form of autism or Asperger's Syndrome? Did he have symptoms which had been overlooked by the community? Was he different? As a child? As an adult? And if Einstein had autism or Asperger's Syndrome, what would that mean in terms of my own child?

These questions led me to Professor Edward Ritvo, world famous physician and researcher in the field of autism. It was with Dr. Ritvo that I came to believe that Einstein did have some form of the syndrome. It was with Dr. Ritvo that I wrote, lectured and later created an audiocassette on the life of Albert Einstein and Autism. And it was with Dr. Ritvo that I came to write and publish *Joey and Sam*, a storybook now sold all over the world, for all children, focusing on autism.

From that work on Albert Einstein as well as the interaction with our son, coupled with an interplay with other parents and their children with the same developmental differences, my early work in social scripting came into being. What began as writing for my own son quickly expanded to writing for others as well as teaching others how to write for their own children and clients. These writing and subsequent speaking engagements brought me into contact with Dr. Andrew Yellen.

Dr. Yellen saw the universal need for this powerful tool. A visionary in his own right, Dr. Yellen perceived how important Social Facilitation would be to those already receiving psychological and educational help, and to all those at risk. He soon invited me to become part of his staff at Yellen and Associates, a large educational and psychological practice with several offices in and around Southern California. As our work together grew it soon became apparent that some sort of written manual for use by practitioners, parents and aides was desperately needed. *Social Facilitation In Action* was created to meet that need. Enjoy!

Illana Katz

Introduction

A youngster, previously diagnosed as having some form of autism, comes to the breakfast table looking a bit disheveled. He seems anxious and annoyed. "Good morning sweetheart," his mother says. There is no reply. The youngster does not even glance at her. He just sits down, fiddles a bit with his table napkin and then stares off into space. A moment later his mother says, "I have something for you."

"What?" he replies, his tone flat, almost as if he is answering while his mind is preoccupied.

She places an envelope in his hands. "I forgot to give this to you last week. It's a card from your Dad and me."

He sits there for a moment, still staring off into space. "Aren't you going to open it?" she asks. He soon looks down at the envelope and slowly begins to open it. He takes out the card, its colorful green cover pleasing to most eyes. He looks at its cover, his face poker flat, and then opens it to read what is written inside. On the left side of the card are three words in his mother's handwriting. YOU ARE WONDERFUL! That's all it says! Yet, those words are like magic. It is like a fairy has suddenly dusted him with happiness. A big grin suddenly appears on his face. His eyes twinkle. He turns toward his mother. She reaches down and gives him a gentle hug. "I love you," she says softly. "I love you too," he replies. It will be a lovely day for him after all.

This is Social Facilitation (SF)!

A child with Asperger's Syndrome is going off to sleep-away camp. He has never been to sleep-away camp before. He is unsure what will happen at camp. With each passing moment his anxiety continues to rise, like a thunderhead letting you know of an impending storm. He begins to pace. A moment later his mother takes out a laminated flyer and hands it to him. On one side of the flyer is a map of the camp. The map shows the location of his tent, the swimming pool, the dining hall, where he can find everything that might interest him and everything that will meet his needs.

On the other side of the flyer is a daily schedule. It tells him what he can expect to happen at camp. It guides him through his day. The schedule tells him what time he will get up in the morning, when he will have breakfast, lunch, dinner and snacks. It informs him when he can go swimming; when he can go horseback riding; and when he can go to archery, arts and crafts, and sports. It tells him when he will have free time and what he can choose to do during that free time. The schedule even leaves room for unexpected changes like special concerts, an overnight campout and field trips. In short, the schedule provides him with the information he will need to prepare himself for a day's events. It provides him with structure and the security of knowing what will come next. It gives him the opportunity to look forward to doing those things he really enjoys and it allows him to plan ahead. What more could he ask?

His pacing soon stops and the child begins to smile. He asks his mother if it is time to put his duffel bag and sleeping bag into the car. He's ready to go!

This is Social Facilitation (SF).

A new family is moving into the house next door. A teenager with special needs watches from an upstairs window as moving van personnel empty their truck, carrying the truck's contents into the house. His mother calls him away from the window. A few minutes later he returns. Each time she calls to him he comes away, only to steadfastly return a few minutes later. He knows something is different. He becomes curious. "Would you like to go next door and meet our new neighbors?" she asks him.

"Yes," he says flatly as he continues to watch. His mother will use this opportunity to help her son strengthen his social skills. She knows that were he to be left to his own devices he would probably go next door, walk in unannounced and say something like, "Mercury is the closest planet to the sun." He might then choose to walk around their house, visually checking out the furniture and boxes. To prevent this inappropriate kind of introduction and behavior she whips out a small writing pad and begins to jot down some words and phrases. As her son continues to gaze out the window she creates what we call a quick script. In this case the quick script will present him with appropriate words and phrases to make this upcoming introduction positive and appropriate.

Within a few minutes she calls him away from the window and sits him down. "Let's go over this together," she says. "When we know what we are going to say, we can go over to the next door neighbor's house and say it. We will be introducing ourselves."

"Okay," he replies. Together they read through the script she has quickly created. She smiles at him and suggests they read it one more time, just for fun. She then has him hold the quick script for a moment as she goes into the kitchen and gets a freshly baked coffee cake from the counter. Together they go next door.

Script in hand, the teenager chooses not to use it but proceeds to introduce himself using the words he has already memorized from the script's contents. He tells the neighbor his name and age and the school he attends. His mother then introduces herself and gives the neighbor the cake she has just baked. The neighbor introduces himself and his family, thanks them for coming and for the lovely cake. He adds that once they are settled he would like to have them come over for a longer visit.

This has been a wonderful opportunity to meet new people and make new friends. It has been socially educational for this teenager. It has been positive and it has been totally appropriate. It can pave the way for other introductions, relationships and potential friendships.

This too is Social Facilitation (SF).

A child with autism enters a crowded room with great trepidation. Within a few moments his external demeanor begins to unravel as the seemingly quiet youngster begins to show signs of anxiety. Head down, he avoids looking at those near him, looking up only fleetingly. Previously holding onto his mother's arm, he lets go, hands now flapping, excitedly emitting odd sounds or repetitive words or phrases. He begins to pace or dance about in some seemingly odd fashion. Unable to cope with the stimulation surrounding him, his behaviors continue to escalate, bringing unwanted attention from others. He is soon removed from the room.

Walking from one class to another a seventh grader at a local middle school sees his friend John, whom he hasn't seen since elementary school. Quickly grabbing John's arm, he then walks up to a third student, one he does not know, and exclaims, "John's here." That student keeps walking, occasionally looking back for a moment, bewildered. The seventh grader, still holding onto John's arm, stops another student and excitedly repeats the same few words, only to get a similar response. All the while John says nothing and seems indifferent. Left unchecked the seventh grader would continue to stop other students on their way to class, never understanding that his excitement at seeing an old friend did not seem to be shared by those with whom he spoke.

A history teacher asks her class a question. One youngster, unable to hold himself back, blurts out an answer as he simultaneously raises his hand. Far from the first time this has happened, the teacher is frustrated at this youngster's repeated failure to follow classroom rules. Cognizant that his scores on intelligence tests are far above the norm, she is also bewildered by his odd answers. She writes herself a note to telephone his parents.

Sitting at his desk, pencil in hand, a fourth grader tries desperately to concentrate on the test that rests before him. Constantly distracted and unable to concentrate, he once again stares off into the distance. His paper is collected, incomplete.

So many things in life appear to be a gamble, a twist in the road, an unexpected detour. Our children are no exception. These little bundles of joy can turn our lives topsy-turvy. They can consume every ounce of emotional, financial and physical strength we have. The frequent calls from the preschool, elementary, and secondary teachers and others can leave us drained and frustrated. Yet, surely these children did not enter these situations hoping to come away with feelings of anxiety or pain or disappointment.

For most of us, deciding to have children involved a whole host of noble, worthy thoughts, projections, dreams and visions. Some of us may have believed ourselves to be master sculptors; powerful beings that would create a blend of ourselves. We would mold a child, teach and guide him. It would be a worthy endeavor, selfless and honorable. And someday, this selfsame child would grow to be another Einstein. Or, so we might have thought!

However, reality can shatter the best of dreams. Perhaps we failed to read some make believe small print in some fairytale contract. If there were such small print, it might have said that there is a contingency of little movers and shakers that moves and shakes to a different rhythm, a unique beat. Even had we read this small print, would we ever have stopped to think that our little bundle might turn out to be one of these little movers and shakers?

The world can be an incredibly complicated place in which to maneuver. As parents and other professionals living and working with developmentally challenged individuals, many of us find ourselves running both their defense and offense, attempting to determine the best environment, the most suitable placement, the perfect setting in which they are best able to both thrive and learn. We collaborate with experts. Sometimes that collaboration can leave us puzzled.

Would a public school setting best meet the needs of this individual at risk or would a private setting be better? Would that individual be better suited to take part in the emotionally challenging environment of the traditional, fully inclusive classroom setting or would he be better off in a separate setting, perhaps even a totally separate campus? Does he require the assistance of a full-time aide, part-time aide or no aide at all? If he does require a classroom aide, should that aide be male or female? These are all important questions to be considered and evaluated.

Just as each individual is unique, so too are the demands, temperament, experience and limitations of a particular instructor or group of instructors. In addition, the kind of material to be mastered coupled with the feelings of that child toward that material needs to play a role in the development of an effective approach. Even factors such as the wallcovering in the classroom, type and intensity of lighting, acoustics and noise level of the class itself are all factors to be considered so that the best placement can be ensured.

So what is Social Facilitation (SF)? Social Facilitation is vital information in visual form. It can provide that key to understanding so desperately lacking in some individuals. With its often crib-note-like form, SF can ease the stress created by new social situations. Use it to increase social understanding. Use it to reduce maladaptive behaviors. Use it to increase practical skills, self-esteem and self-confidence. It can be an enormously powerful tool. Harness its power and open up the world to the many whom we love and serve.

The manual you now hold focuses on a fascinating approach to help people with varying developmental differences and difficulties. It is an approach that may help them function at their best in the least restrictive and most comprehensive environment. It provides a means by which others can help them better understand the world around them. Using a group of techniques we lump together under this name we call Social Facilitation, it is our belief that many individuals diagnosed with some form of autism, Asperger's

Syndrome, Tourette Syndrome, Obsessive Compulsive Disorder, Attention Deficit Disorder, and other learning disabilities and behavioral difficulties, can increase their ability to understand, respond and function more confidently and appropriately in the real world.

Social Facilitation can be equally valid and useful in academic settings, at home, out in the community and on vacation. Through the various types of social scripting available in SF, it is our goal to give you the ability to design and create effective quick scripts, stories, albums, and adventures for those at risk. As the techniques you use are employed on a regular basis, it is our belief that a more receptive, happier, more contented, enthusiastic individual will greet you each day.

PART I

Chapter I

Old Paradigms for New

Toronto, Canada was a lovely place for an International Autism Convention. It was abuzz with excitement as new ideas were put forth. Yet, it would be an event following the conference which would transform and reshape my understanding of the potentials that may lie hidden under the umbrella of pervasive developmental disorders.

With the conference coming to a close many of us had chosen to spend a day aboard a tour bus headed for Niagara Falls and towns between. It was a lovely day in July. Perfect weather. Perfect air. Magnificent surroundings. Old and young, disabled and abled boarded the bus, some strolling down the aisles, some lumbering along, finding seats, stowing packages, snacks, and other goodies. The bus quickly filled to capacity, people chattering, greeting friends of a few days. The chattering grew louder as people settled aboard, a busload of tired but otherwise contented conference participants and family members set free from days of lively lectures, discussions and exchanges, their heads now stuffed with new ideas and updated information. The new information would now mingle with the old, re-package and re-integrate itself, so that new outlooks and perspectives would carve themselves into a new gestalt.

We settled back into padded seats anxiously anticipating the day's distractions and rewards. Toronto had been glorious, the people warm and friendly. We had become a sort of family unit; and though one row of bus passengers may not have known the specific life experiences of the next, we were all the same. We were linked by an umbrella of neurological and psychological aberration and concern.

Over those few days a camaraderie had quite naturally developed amongst the hundreds and hundreds of participants. Knowing, accepting, feeling, sharing, there was no need for apologies when a child or adult had a problem; we had all been there. There was no need for specifics; our lives were variations on a theme.

My mind drifted back to the bus, which now seemed to let out a sigh as it inched forward, leaving the hotel behind, walling off a chapter in time. As the day's adventure got underway, I suddenly became aware that my seat seemed to be moving, rhythmically rocking. Instinctively knowing that it was not a tire on the bus going flat, I turned around. Behind me sat a man who appeared to be in his early fifties. Seated beside him was a somewhat more elderly woman, his mother. The gentleman was rocking back and forth, back and forth, repeating the same sort of mantra over and over, almost melodically. "Ha, ha, ha," he said, "I'm a good boy, I'm a good boy." There would be silence for a few moments while he continued to rhythmically rock, and then the entire word and behavioral sequence would repeat itself.

We made a few selected stops on the way to the falls, getting on and off the bus. We saw the falls and went to dinner. Whether by coincidence or design, this same gentleman and his mother were seated at our table. Introductions were made. My husband and I spoke to his mother about the conference, autism and family. We discovered that, even though we lived a thousand miles apart, we seemed to know many of the same people. The mother told me that her son was one of the first children ever given the diagnosis of autism by Dr. Leo Kanner. Here was a mother who had lived it all.

Dinners were ordered. Time passed and no dinners arrived. I could not help but notice how often this mother gazed down at her wristwatch. She finally disclosed to me how important food was to her son and how necessary it was that it be served at a specific time. That time had long since passed.

I quickly glanced at her son, noting a change in his demeanor. The once peaceful, withdrawn gentlemen had been replaced. Having initially been quiet and fairly immobile, he was now humming and rocking. Within another minute or two he began to hit himself on the head with one hand while biting himself on the other, his humming growing louder as each minute passed.

I watched closely as his mother took a blank envelope and pen from her purse. On the envelope she quickly wrote the following, "Dinner will be here in ten minutes." To see her write for him, as if he were able to read, stopped me dead in my tracks. Could this be so? Could one who appeared to be severely afflicted by the syndrome of autism read? And not only read, but understand and appropriately respond? The mother handed the envelope to her son. He took it, seemed to read it, folded it in half and placed it in his pocket.

Like a billowing storm suddenly subdued, there was an immediate and profound change in this man's behavior. The biting, hitting and rocking ceased. The humming was gone. Once again he sat peacefully. Yes, he had read it. And from his response he clearly understood it. Furthermore, he was able to reestablish self-control. Whoa!

I got up and ran to the nearest waiter informing him that if dinner did not arrive in the next few minutes, chaos would. The waiter must have believed me because he was at our table, food in hand, before I was.

How often do we pass judgment upon others based solely on what we perceive their limitations to be? How often do appearances fail to reveal the person within? And how could we engage the person within so that his true abilities could be tapped and used to foster repeated and varied reciprocal social interaction?

Our own young son, then perhaps only six years old, spoke quite well, by comparison to this gentleman. I had been writing for him using what I would later call quick scripts, since before he was age five. If our son was labeled high functioning because he could speak clearly by age three, even if his vocabulary was limited, what set him apart from this man? The ability to understand was there for each of them. It seemed to be, in part, a matter of how easily we could get to it, foster and encourage its use. What if the only thing separating this man, our son, and so many others was a knowing soul trapped in a non-compliant body? How many others were like this gentleman? How many others were somewhere between him and our son?

My thoughts ran wild, letting loose a veritable torrent of interpolations, each one building upon the preceding, each one yielding a striking human potential previously unimaginable, except perhaps in dreams.

The breathtaking beauty of Niagara Falls had been memorable, but the rumble and wake left by this chance encounter between mother and son was an awakening, a rebirth, an experiential reevaluation, a revelation. My understanding of autism and human potential would never be the same.

Glancing up at mother and son as we ate, I smiled. They seemed to have such a beautifully symbiotic relationship. She thanked me and proceeded to describe their life together. That picture revealed a son who shopped with her, organized the cupboards at home, kept the house spotless; a son who would hand her ingredients as she cooked, even prior to her asking for them; a son who was her constant companion. That's what he really was, you know, her companion.

My mind drifted to my son, to the many sons and daughters we all hold so dear. How many of these children, our children, our students, our clients, were reading, and we didn't know? How many understood far more than we gave them credit for knowing? I had known that our own youngster with autism was reading some words between ages three and four, certainly long before he could ask for a drink of water. How many others had developed this same skill without our ever having been aware?

Harking back to the convention just ended, there had been a panel discussion hosted by several young adults with autism. One such young person, a young man who had recently graduated with honors from Yale University, related his life story to us. His story included his relating to the audience the fact that though he didn't say a word until he was past age five, he was reading the newspaper over the side of his crib by eighteen months. Reading the newspaper over the side of the crib by eighteen months?

Snapping back to attention at the dinner table with this gentleman and his mother I began to connect the dots. What if our son, the Yale graduate and this gentleman at dinner were not an exception at all? What if a sizable percentage of these people had somehow developed the ability to decode written words long before they spoke? How could we help to set free a mind held hostage behind some stone wall? How could that wall be scaled?

If indeed the visual arena is the key, if it is one of untapped ability, then why not use that ability? Why not harness that strength? Tears welled up in my eyes. Visually, came the answer within. VISUALLY! Oh, my God! VISUALLY!

Chapter II

Young Albert Einstein

Say the name Albert Einstein and what is the first thing that comes to mind? $E = MC^2$? Theory of Relativity? Father of Modern Physics? An old man with white hair? Someone who spoke with a thick foreign accent? An eccentric? A genius?

Now picture a young Albert Einstein, a child, a youngster born in Bavaria, a part of Germany, way back in 1879. Can you see him in your mind's eye? And if so, isn't he the one we'd probably picture as a child prodigy, or at least a most precocious bouncing baby boy? If so, think again! Albert Einstein appears to have been anything but gifted as a child, teenager, or young adult! His development appears to have been very uneven. And, in fact, he might have appeared to any of us today as particularly odd, developmentally different, perhaps even Asperger-like or mildly autistic, if not a high-functioning autistic youngster! Just ask Dr. Edward Ritvo, world-renowned researcher and physician in the field of autism and Professor Emeritus, University of California, Los Angeles.

As a small child Albert Einstein's parents thought he was sub-normal. His grandmother would refer to him as a "dullard," his relatives regarded him as a black sheep in the family, his nurse referred to him as "Father Bore" and many others just considered him rather dull. Albert Einstein was slow in learning to speak and respond; and it is said that even at the age of nine years, his language skills were remarkably limited. When not having a tantrum he appeared to be quite sedentary, disliking physical activity. Young Einstein was silent and solitary. He had no friends. It is said that throughout life he would relate best to his sister Maja.

Young Albert did not like crowds and noise. As a youngster, parades would cause him to flee. He played with few toys. He was backward, prone to severe tantrums and withdrawn from the world.

His limited fluency in his mother tongue provided difficulty for him as he entered school. He continued to have no friends. He was slow working and solitary. He seemed to have difficulty forming any kind of relationship with any children other than his younger sister. His teachers believed him to have had absolutely no special skills or talents, leading many to believe that he would never amount to anything.

However, Albert Einstein liked books. He liked to read, on his own, at his own pace. He liked to read books about things that he found interesting. They were tools to learn about the world. Books revealed how things worked and how people functioned. They helped him learn to adapt to a world in which he did not seem to fit. Books were effective and efficient tools for understanding. What appeared in print gave him a framework by which to relate to those around him. Books were his lifeline to appropriate and acceptable societal interaction. They facilitated his social, emotional and educational interaction. And, throughout his life, books would provide him with a comfortable and comforting way of learning, of adapting, of interacting.

When a family friend gave Einstein a book on philosophy he gobbled it up, learning all he could about the subject. When required by the educational system to study religion he appears to have become a veritable religious fanatic. Books modified even his dietary habits. When immersed in religious study he became intensely ritualistic and would compose songs in honor of God, songs that he sang to himself on his way to school.

His religious fascination continued until the age of twelve when he was given his first geometry book. Fascinated by the book he abandoned religion to study geometry, calling this book his "Holy Geometry Book," and becoming totally immersed and involved in its content.

Einstein appears to have learned on his own, in his own way, in an environment that met his needs. Indeed, one might say he had a habit or style of serial preoccupations that became evident during his school years. Perhaps we might say that he perseverated on anything that interested him to the exclusion of what others thought.

Throughout his teens Einstein's social difficulties continued. Teachers found his behavior in class to be disruptive and peculiar. Years later Einstein himself would agree that his presence in school held others back. Appearing depressed and nervous he would be expelled from his secondary school.

Yet his mother, supported by extended family's money, would find a way to have him admitted to a private school in Switzerland where he could complete his secondary education. Though these new surroundings would prove to be more conducive to his needs, class attendance would continue to be difficult for him.

His aberrant classroom behavior continued to be an obstacle for him as his classmates found him to be distant and uncaring. They took notice of his frequent need to pace. Some of them would comment on his unique ability to disappear into himself, his appearance of withdrawing from the world.

When Einstein later attended university, his personal peculiarities continued to haunt him. He failed to follow directions, would often balk at his need to attend class and to study what was required of him by his instructors. His behavior in the laboratory was unacceptable and sometimes even dangerous to himself. He is described as having failed to listen to anything or anyone and was considered by some in authority to be downright lazy.

His classmates considered him pedantic and a source of peculiar personal advice, talking incessantly to an individual one day yet hardly seeming to know him the next. Like his earlier serial preoccupations with religion and geometry, Einstein would now perseverate on physics. He was hopelessly impractical, could not manage money, and was unable to make up his mind even about simple, everyday matters. He would agree with whomever he spoke with last. It is said, in fact, that, had he not been taken under wing by a few students, who would invest limitless time and energy working tirelessly with him, Albert Einstein might never have completed his formal education nor given us the benefit of his great genius.

Without question, Albert Einstein's work in physics may be some of the most important in the twentieth century. Einstein learned through the written word. The written word was his best connection to this world. It was his pillar of strength. We believe it can be a pillar of strength to those whose needs we serve. If Einstein had some form of developmental difficulty, and achieved all he did, then those we work with and love deserve no less. Many an Einstein could be out there. We believe the written word to be the necessary link to their emergence.

Chapter III

The Word and the Flow

Characters on paper can take on a life of their own. Ask any novelist! Characters can interact in ways never dreamed of, leaving an author scrambling to jot down their words and actions, even if those words and actions are not what was in mind for those characters. Sounds crazy. Nonetheless, it happens.

Ideas may shape our words, but the opposite is true as well. Words have an impact on our ability to express or modify our ideas. Ideas attached to words can pop into the conscious mind to be snapped up, evaluated, and accepted or rejected. And you begin to wonder what came first, the word or the idea?

Yet, we have only to glance at the Bible, and specifically the Old Testament, to gain insight into the relationship of words and ideas. Open the work to its very first pages and what do we read? Light. Let there be light. Before the reality of light itself there was the word. The reality of LIGHT took shape based upon the WORD! WORD first, REALITY second.

By extension then we might ask, *if there is no word, is there a reality*? Well, *is there*? What would happen if we had no vocabulary, no language of any sort, shared or idiopathic, group or individual, to define what we experience? How might we respond to a world filled with nameless, moving, undefined stimuli; a world in which we were on the outside looking in, a world in which we were unprepared to play a part, did not have a clue how to play a part, or did not even understand we had a part to play?

In such a world, might we feel left out, alone, lonely, and/or abandoned? Might not this be our worst nightmare? And, isn't it possible that given this set of circumstances, we might respond in much the same way that many people with autism, Asperger's Syndrome and other developmental disabilities frequently do?

The journey of those we seek to help is a complex one. Yet, if we are to succeed we need to reach out and bridge the gap between them and the world, no matter how wide, no matter how deep. And, perhaps, if we work together, we can make a difference in their lives and ours as well. Let us give them the tools for understanding. Let us give them the props, the roles, the meanings that they deserve, that they so desperately need. Let us give them a box full of life's tools; tools that they can take from place to place. Let us provide the connection, the WORD!

Daniel Goleman in his powerfully written book *Emotional Intelligence* talks about words and their impact when he refers to a problem some individuals have that would seem to be unrelated to those whose needs we are serving. And yet, his words and ideas spill over, providing us with some guidance.

Mr. Goleman refers to a disability called *alexithymia,* an inability to find and/or use words to define an emotion, something we often face with the many individuals we serve. Dr. Peter Sifnewos, a Harvard psychiatrist, coined the term in 1972. Dr. Sifnewos said that those who fit the definition "Give the impression of being different, alien beings, having come from an entirely different world, living in the midst of a society, which is dominated by feelings" (pg. 50). According to Goleman, it is not that alexithymics don't feel anything, but are, instead, unable to recognize or understand what they are feeling. Simply put, they lack self-awareness. What would we do if we could feel but were unable to identify our feelings? What if we were unable to discriminate between tolerance, suffering, endurance, sympathy, empathy, love, or respect? What if inspiration, affection, fanaticism and passion were unrecognized, just words with nowhere to go? What if we could not understood these emotions? And if we were not able to recognize these things in ourselves how could we recognize them in others?

Is it any wonder then, that when people who suffer from alexithymia are moved to feel something, the experience can be so overwhelming and baffling that they avoid it?

Yet, what does the word alexithymia have to do with the population we are confronting? What if you processed information in a different manner, or a slower speed than the majority of the rest of the population? What if your processing skills were so limited that you almost needed to see things in slow motion to absorb them? What if you missed out on a third or more of everything that went on around you so that the world seemed to be a confusing, anxiety-producing assault on your every thought, your every move? Wouldn't this processing problem affect your ability to understand appropriate interactions between self and other? If we were unable to understand a social situation in motion, if we were unable to keep pace with others, the world would be a most confusing and frightening place. Within a social situation, if we had limited reference points and few internal definitions to draw upon, how might we respond?

We believe individuals at risk can develop the understanding necessary to adapt more comfortably and appropriately to many social situations. However, without some form of educational adaptations appropriate to their unique learning style, many of the individuals we seek to help might appear to be similar to those suffering from alexithymia.

When Goleman refers to those with alexithymia, it almost sounds as if he is referring to those with some form of PDD or autism. "Feelings come to them, when they come at all, as a befuddling bundle of distress." He believes those suffering from alexithymia are not only unable to identify, recognize or understand feelings, but, because of this inability to individually discriminate between the many discrete emotional terms, they are unable to put their feelings into words, and therefore, are unable to connect to them.

When Goleman refers to those he defines with alexithymia perhaps he is giving us clues to understanding our children, clients and others with needs. Simply put, he is saying that if someone doesn't have either an internal visual picture label or word label to hang a particular emotion upon, he can neither recognize that emotion as a discrete entity to help himself nor understand another.

For example, without an internal understanding of specific emotional terms like suffering, tolerance, love, and empathy, how could an individual understand and identify those same emotions in others? How could he recognize them, either consciously or unconsciously, in others so that he might relate, respond, or share how he feels about their situation? These are significant statements, statements that may tell us a great deal about our youngsters and clients in need. Goleman's words may give us clues about those we seek to help. His words help us understand what subjects need to be addressed within the various forms of Social Facilitation we may choose to use. For example, if we can provide information vital to understanding, label and define it, place it in an appropriate framework, and give it a familiar setting, the individual might be better able to internalize and accept it. Having then made it a part of his experience, he might then be better able to begin to use it appropriately and comfortably.

In his book Goleman goes on to provide us with a possible way to lift the burdens of confusion and frustration that those he speaks about confront each day. He makes use of a concept called *flow,* a term defined previously by Michaly Csikszentmihalyi.

Csikszentmihalyi says that when people are involved in activities that effortlessly capture and hold their attention the brain 'quiets down' allowing them to try a more difficult task.

Haven't you ever felt that there are places in which you feel more comfortable? Haven't you ever found that you are most relaxed, calm or serene in a particular place; somewhere in your home, or a place like a backyard garden, or a particular place in a library, or a cozy spot in a book store? More than likely an individual at risk also has a spot or two that could allow him to feel less vulnerable, less overwhelmed, more able to relax and attempt to better learn and interact. "The flow refers to that state between being bored and anxious. Flow is internal and exemplifies a moment where the individual is doing something that is perfectly balanced to their needs, holding their attention yet failing to cause stress or anxiety," says Csikszentmihalyi.

When a young child repeatedly reviews a picture book, studying its pages, scrutinizing each scene quietly, he may be in the flow. When a teenager is nestled quietly in a beanbag chair, his head buried in a book, he may be in the flow. When Albert Einstein studied his "Holy Geometry" book, he may have been in the flow. Each of these people may have found those areas in which they could feel at peace, safe, comfortable and able to learn, that place of the flow.

I sometimes tell people, tongue in cheek, that if their two-year-old youngster prefers books to toys, taking them to bed instead of stuffed animals; if that same two-year-old craves the television show "Wheel of Fortune," watch out, he or she may be developing a bit differently. Though meant to be humorous, perhaps this statement isn't so far out! How many of us were aware that many of these children knew words or phrases on sight before age four, yet referred to themselves as "you"? How many of us were aware of other early differences?

Why focus on the visual? Because it can be an area of flow. Because the visual may hold the key to opening the door that separates us. Many of these youngsters seem fascinated by letters, words and numbers. It appears that through letters, words and numbers they can unlock the secrets of the world around them. Combined with pictures and squiggles they begin to understand what may have previously been inaccessible to them. Letters combined to yield words. Words combined to yield phrases. Letters and words and phrases and pictures all providing understanding.

In light of Goleman's work and what we already know about feelings and what we believe to be their importance to words, "feeling" type words need to be carefully chosen to succinctly reflect that emotion. Together we can help them accomplish what would be difficult, if not impossible, for them to accomplish on their own.

In the book *Reading Too Soon*, author Susan Martins Miller writes about hyperlexic children, defined by her as those children with a precocious ability to read, difficulty in processing spoken language, and abnormal social skills. She believes "Wheel of Fortune" is a favorite because "letters turn into words and a big, colorful spinning wheel - what more could they ask for? Hyperlexic children just cannot stop themselves. They love visual stimulation. They read everything in sight. They will read everything from cereal boxes, traffic signs, fast-food menus, newspaper headlines, advertising slogans, aisle markers in the grocery store, toy packages, scoreboards, whatever happens to be there. They just cannot stop themselves. They just love visual stimulation. Parents sometimes wish their children could pay as much attention to other areas as they do to visual stimulation," she says.

While I agree that the children love the visual stimulation of "Wheel of Fortune," and agree that I wish the children could pay as much attention to other areas as they do to visual stimulation, it is precisely this visual excitement and interest on their part that gives us the impetus to use Social Facilitation. Even Daniel Goleman says that many individuals can learn to read a social situation. Whether he means that statement literally is debatable. However, we do. Later in this manual we will demonstrate how Social Facilitation techniques can meet this challenge; for if a word can be used as a vehicle to express how an individual feels, if a written word can enhance understanding or reduce anxiety, then it is the word that may bring about change.

Chapter IV

"SPAIR" versus "SWAIR"

It has been said that we change every day. Cells die and new cells are born. We are not exactly the same person today as yesterday. We have changed. But we have changed more than just physically. Each day, in fact each moment, we take in new information and integrate it with preexisting information. We then modify our data bank, so to speak. In this way, we are somehow continuously recreated into a slightly different being. In addition to our daily physical changes then, each of us is constantly changing intellectually, emotionally, behaviorally and socially as well.

Experientially, we take in new information each moment. This new information goes through a series of hoops and loops which we shall call "SPAIR." We use the term "SPAIR" as an acronym to better explain how we take in information, moment by moment, and are modified by it.

You might say, "SPAIR" me, SPAIR standing for:

S Stimulus (internal or external)

P Perception (physical senses, including feelings)

A Analysis (bank of information to which all incoming stimuli are compared for a response)

I Integration (modifying of old information to accommodate new data and appropriate placement of new data)

R Response (action taken, could be physical, verbal, emotional or internal)

Having made it through all the hoops and loops, the information is then integrated with preexisting knowledge so that a newly modified understanding of the world takes place.

The world is in a constant state of change. It changes and we change. We change and the world changes. We probably don't think about these changes, but the relationship is interactive. Together, we are in sync.

However, some individuals are out of sync with the world around them. They don't seem to integrate data very well and they fall behind. Perhaps the data takes too long to become assimilated; or perhaps pieces of data taken in are disconnected or disjointed, much like a jigsaw puzzle resting on a table with no one to arrange and connect the pieces. Other individuals find it difficult to accept new data at all, blocking the stimulus from even entering, withdrawing at the mere hint of it. Still others seem to be able to accept and integrate the data to a greater or lesser extent, perhaps only at a slower processing speed.

We are not just talking about the recognition and integration of macro change, the kind of change that takes place as the result of going on a vacation or some special journey. We are talking about the little, tiny changes that occur continuously, every moment of every day ... changes that can result from reading the morning newspaper or watching a television program or engaging in conversation. We are talking about the kind of change that occurs when we eat or drink or ride a bike, walk or swim – constant, continuous change.

If I see you today I am one person. When I see you tomorrow, I will be a bit different, and so will you, and so will the world around us, all having taken in new information and been modified by it, whether we wanted to or not. As individuals we receive some kind of stimulus, we perceive it, we analyze it, we integrate it, are changed by it and can respond appropriately.

For most individuals the "SPAIR" model works well. We meet someone on the street and learn they are related to a neighbor or friend. Shortly thereafter we are invited to that friend or neighbor's home. When we visit the neighbor the acquaintance is there. Having already integrated the new data with the old, we respond appropriately and knowledgeably to neighbor and acquaintance.

However, given the same situation for individuals with developmental or learning difficulties and without benefit of some type of SF, social problems often become apparent. They become apparent because of the variation in our "SPAIR" model. This difficulty would arise specifically in the areas following the "S" of the stimulus. While the area of stimulus seems to be intact and is usually perceived by the individual, it is in the area of perception and all that comes after that, that the difficulties seem to arise. It is here that the breakdown begins to occur.

One day I watched as a six year old child, previously diagnosed with a more mild form of autism, was given the task of arranging a puzzle which, when completed, would reveal the face of a happy youngster with features and hair. His mission would be to put together the ten or twelve puzzle pieces, to integrate the pieces into a meaningful whole. What might seem a simple task to most youngsters was a total mystery to this child. The young boy could not seem to arrange or connect the pieces in any meaningful way. The eyes, eyebrows, nose, mouth, skin, hair, and so on, remained disjointed and meaningless to the child. When asked about the pieces separately, the youngster could identify the eyes, ears, etc. as well as the use of each element, yet could not connect the pieces into an integrated whole. It was as if the individual features were concrete, freestanding objects.

For this child the SPAIR model does not work. Instead he seems to operate under a pseudo form of SPAIR, which we could call SWAIR. In this model only the "S", the initial stimulus, remains the same. It is in the very next letter, the "P" of perception that his difficulties began to arise. Here the "P" perception has deteriorated into "W" – withdrawal, resulting in the model going awry. If the individual at risk functions at this level and withdraws here, following many stimuli, how then might the balance of the acronym function? What would ultimately be its outcome? Perhaps the stimulus remains so isolated, so concrete and rigid, its edges so defined that it will have no seeming value at that point in time. Like an eyeball in the jigsaw puzzle above, it remains simply an eyeball and not part of a face. Perhaps the individual is able to somehow connect the eyeball, even if it appears in the wrong place so that some type of analysis, integration and response might be possible. SF can be introduced at any point in the processing sequence. As an intervention, it is often used as a preemptive measure, especially when it is known that an individual does not have any understanding or experience with some upcoming situation or project; or when it is known that the individual is easily agitated, frustrated and prone to act out in an unproductive manner.

Nothing is written in concrete. An SF story delivered prior to the event could help the individual successfully complete a task; however, it would have failed to give the individual the full opportunity to "figure it out on his own." Sometimes, however, we have little choice. To intervene prior to the event or wait for the SPAIR/SWAIR to begin to break down is truly a judgment call and depends upon the individual and the situation at hand.

When we employ SF along the SPAIR, as needed, we have the opportunity to see where the process breaks down. In this case, just as we would not take antibiotics before the body has an infection, we would not have used SF before there is a breakdown in SPAIR. We could then continue to stand back and allow the process to continue, ultimately unsuccessfully, of course; or, we could choose to intervene. As much as we are able, taking this individual, with his needs, into consideration, an attempt was made to allow him the opportunity to resolve the problem without stepping in. And, as in other cases, the choice was ours. In this example the child continued to the puzzle's completion, never amending his error, the result being a rejection of the finished product.

Social Facilitation has its effects at various stages of the SPAIR/SWAIR process. It can be used between the administration of the stimulus "S" and the withdrawal "W" of the individual, helping prevent the individual from becoming overwhelmed and subject to withdrawal. It can be introduced between the "W" of withdrawal and the "A" of analysis, so that if the individual has not found it necessary to withdraw, SF can provide a basis of analysis. SF can be introduced between the "A" of analysis and the "I" of integration because it can take the old and new information and make it mesh. For it is here that information may be held in abeyance, disconnected from understanding and usefulness and disconnected from integration and response. It is here that the individual often becomes almost locked up in a kind of concrete "sameness," locked up in limbo. Finally, SF can be injected between the "I" of integration and the "R" of response so that when everything else is in place, the appropriate response is the result.

Most of us have heard the quick little saying, "Garbage in – garbage out." In this case we can easily see how the misperception of a stimulus could easily result in a totally confusing, disjointed and ultimately frustrating experience.

I heard a story not long ago about a special young man, previously diagnosed as being in the autism/Asperger's spectrum. The young man's family was quite friendly with the family in the next home. One day, the family in the next home bought a new computer, one with all the latest bells and whistles. The young man's family went next door for a few minutes before dinner to see the new computer. They soon left and returned home.

About midnight, the next-door neighbors heard a noise in the room where they had just set up their new computer. Quietly they arose out of their bed. Grabbing hold of a heavy object, the man and his wife tiptoed into the adjacent room. When they clicked on the light, who should they find but the boy from next door. He was busily working away on the computer. Needless to say, his appearance was both unwelcome and unsettling. The neighbors were very upset, and rightly so. They had thought an intruder was in their home. The young man's presence was not appropriate. In fact, had they not recognized him, he might have been hurt. When the parents were telephoned to come and get their son they found him reluctant to leave. He had been happily working away and could not understand why his presence was a problem. The displeasure of all concerned was a complete mystery to him. In his eyes, the computer was part of his world and as such his need to make use of it was only natural. When he hears the word "computer" put with next door neighbor and with his limited understanding of social norms, limited understanding of social boundaries, feelings and empathy, his natural analysis says that the computer has no owner and has only to be gathered to self. It is therefore always available. This new information may or may not have been integrated in a cohesive data bank. Therefore, the outcome is random. In this case his response was swift and immediate. He left his home, walked to the neighbor's house, opened the front door, found the room in which the computer was set up, turned it on and began to play. His presence was met with rejection.

Yet, this child was in no way being aggressive, nor was he maliciously breaking into the neighbor's home. The computer was merely part of the environment from which he reaches out and pulls toward himself. There is no discrete separation between him and it. With the use of Social Facilitation, a quick script, story , album, or adventure could quickly be created to meet his needs prior to this kind of incident. It would be introduced prior to a problem, preventing a breakdown in the SPAIR model.

In the case of a family where a child is not developmentally delayed or disabled, the child would have understood social mores. He would have known that personal belongings, including the neighbor's home, are sacrosanct. He would have waited until the following day before going next door. He would have knocked on the door and asked permission to see the new computer. And, in most instances, he would have gained access to it.

We have only to employ Social Facilitation at the appropriate moment to set the SPAIR model back on track. Obviously, it isn't always possible to catch every potential problem prior to its appearance, but the more we create and use these types of scripting to preempt a problem, the more likely that eventually there could be associations between one kind of event and another so that more generalizations and extrapolations become possible. If we can insert SF to help the individual adjust his perception to what the majority of society would deem appropriate, then his analysis, integration and subsequent responses might appear to be more within agreed upon, appropriate levels.

In a world of constant stimulus and change, in essence, SF is a kind of a prop, bridging the two models and helping put the individual at risk back on the SPAIR model.

Putting the SPAIR/SWAIR model into practical action, we view the preceding story as follows:

SPAIR–SWAIR CHART

SPAIR MODEL Non-disabled individual (not at risk)	**SWAIR MODEL** LD/PDD/Asperger's/Autism (at risk)
Stimulus	**S**timulus
Perception Understands social norms Understands social boundaries Understands feelings Is empathetic	**W**ithdrawal Limited understanding of social norms Limited understanding of social boundaries Limited understanding of feelings Limited empathy
Analysis Personal belongings including house are to be respected (not used without permission)	**A**nalysis Belongings have no owner and are therefore always available
Integration Databank of old information is integrated with new information, including stimulus	**I**ntegration New information may or may not be integrated into a cohesive databank; therefore, outcome is random

Response

Knock
Ask permission
at an appropriate time of day

Response

Use without permission
at any time, day or night

End Result (Societal Views and Understanding)

Acceptance

Rejection

Chapter V

All the World's a Stage

Oftentimes, fiction can point to something useful in the real world. Even a make believe story or film can, unknowingly, shed new light on something or trigger some new idea. For our use, a Hollywood film entitled "City of Angels" may have provided such a clue.

One of the main protagonists in this film is an angel named Seth, an empathetic, gentle, sweet, innocent creature who develops a particular interest in a female surgeon. Having a somewhat limited understanding of humanity, he is terribly naive. In addition he has had no direct experience and no comprehension of the sense of touch, taste or smell.

Dressed in black and making his home in the public library Seth is a kind of messenger/chauffeur in the film. His job is to meet people when they die and take them to wherever dead people go. When not greeting people, he is free to roam the earth, socializing with fellow angels and observing humanity.

On one of Seth's assignments, while waiting for an upcoming human to pass on, he becomes intrigued with the physical and emotional efforts of a particular doctor to save her patient. Having witnessed the doctor's despair, frustrations and guilt at her own inability to save her patient's life, he becomes intrigued by her behavior. Though choosing to remain invisible to the doctor he begins to follow her around. At this point we, the audience, begin to wonder if Seth's interest in this physician is purely to find a way to help her understand her limitations, or to help himself better understand humanity and his own limitations based on lack of direct experience.

At one point Seth accompanies the surgeon to a fruit market where she picks up a pear (a prop) and smells it; something many of us might do. Seth, in turn, picks up a cactus (a prop) and smells it; something many of us might consider a bit unusual. Why? What made the doctor's behavior appropriate and Seth's behavior inappropriate? Or is it inappropriate?

Let's spend a moment and focus on the props themselves, the pear and the cactus. What is a prop? By definition, a prop is any inanimate or animate object which assists in the understanding of a scene or any social situation. Props can be people, animals, foods, plants, books, furniture, etc.

Use of any prop can seem totally appropriate, somewhat appropriate, somewhat inappropriate or totally inappropriate. You and I might agree that any prop might have a single use or multiple uses. Scratching your back with a gun might not be appropriate, but defending yourself with one might. The appearance of a surgeon entering the operating theatre dressed in a bathing suit, fins and snorkel would certainly be considered inappropriate. Yet, the appearance of that same surgeon similarly dressed and jumping off a boat to observe and enjoy flora and fauna in the ocean depths would be considered totally appropriate.

This shared view of appropriate versus inappropriate use of props can also be subtle. If one were to jump into the ocean in shark-infested waters during a hurricane, you and I would agree that this behavior was not only inappropriate, but reckless.

Taking this a bit farther, if you scratch your head with your own hand, thus turning your hand into a prop, that's appropriate! What if you scratch your head using your neighbor's hand, turning their hand into a prop? This, of course is equally inappropriate!

Scratching your back with a plastic back-scratcher (prop) – appropriate; scratching your back with a tooth brush (prop) – somewhat inappropriate; scratching your back with a Q tip – totally inappropriate. Notice how we start getting into some very subtle changes, changes that can open us up to scrutiny and ridicule by others.

What is appropriate and inappropriate is often influenced by group mores and customs, societal variation, ethnic differences, family values and individual beliefs. And all too often the distinctions between what is appropriate versus inappropriate can be very, very subtle. What may appear inappropriate to me may appear totally appropriate to you.

Finding a way to teach individuals with limited social understanding of these shades of gray which may change with exposure to varying cultures and countries, can make our job even more difficult, but not insurmountable.

Our props in the supermarket scene above (pear and cactus) can point to more than the problem of appropriate and inappropriate. We often decide on the purchase of something edible, like a piece of fruit, by its texture, its smell or both. From my own background a cactus is a funny-looking, prickly plant found in desert regions. Cacti have no discernable use other than one's need to avoid their painful touch. On the other hand, a pear is a sweet, edible, fruit.

Within the film "City of Angels" was Seth's use of the cactus inappropriate? Yes! Why? Because, in addition to my understanding of cacti as being non-edible, his behavior served no functional use. Seth was incapable of feeling its touch, responding to its taste or sampling its smell. He was mimicking a similar behavior being used by another life form, behavior that would give him no information, no further understanding.

However, what might seem inappropriate to one observer whose experience with a cactus suggests a very limited use – pot it and water it, avoid its touch – may not be so clear to someone of another culture who might actually make use of cacti in some kind of recipe. Without an understanding of a greater cacti, an observer could find fault in the behavior of another when in actuality it is the judgment of the observer that is the problem.

In reality, there are those who enjoy eating cactus and who prepare it in a myriad of ways. Certain ethnic groups apparently prepare it from fresh varieties, others buy it canned. Seth's behavior may have been inappropriate, but not for the reasons some may have thought.

The point being made is that many children and adults with developmental differences may have no understanding or very limited understanding of a particular prop and therefore may respond unfavorably if the prop is used in an unfamiliar way. Many of these individuals hold rigid beliefs about particular props so that the use of these props in new situations is confusing and anxiety producing. And, whereas the bulk of society can rapidly adjust to an old prop with a new or expanded use, to provide our developmentally different population with the tools to more easily make this adjustment is a bit more complex, but not impossible, merely requiring a unique approach: that of SF.

Social Facilitation can concretely show appropriate use or multiple uses of a prop. How?

- Keep a small dictionary with you whenever possible.

- Frequently refer to that dictionary for multi-use definitions of a given word or phrase.

- Check out the many possible uses and definitions for a prop whose use and meaning is not readily understood by the individual.

- Be aware of the use of that prop within other contexts that may or may not lend themselves to the scenario in which you are attempting to increase social understanding.

- Let flexibility in the face of rigid beliefs help guide you as you prepare some type of social tool for the individual in need.

- Try to shape understanding, while allowing for a fluidity or growth of a term, word or concept.

- Always keep in mind, goals can change, they are often fluid. What is important is a solid foundation and a dependable structure.

The film we have used thus far can lend itself to our use a bit more. Take another prop; tears. Within the setting of the film our protagonist could see tears, but could not taste them, smell them, nor touch them. To him, tears were a visual expression, the result of an excess of emotion felt by the human body. As an angel he was aware of how the body manufactured tears as well as when and why they came into use. Like many individuals with developmental differences and disabilities, Seth did not experientially understand the emotion behind the tears, but only understood them as a response to some kind of stimulus or set of stimuli.

How might an individual with some form of autism or other pervasive developmental disorder respond to tears? Given the desire, the individual could certainly see them, touch them, taste them and even smell them. He might also know how and why a body generates tears physiologically. But he might be unable to comprehend the anguish of another human being separate from himself, nor understand the circumstances that produced that anguish when he was not part of it.

Before the development of any kind of story, quick script, album or adventure, the facilitator needs, of course, to understand the limitations of the individual at risk. His work will include the personalizing of the information regarding the prop, what it's for and why. The facilitator needs to find a way to make this learning process safe and comforting. The facilitator needs to be relaxed, at ease. It is important to find something already understood, already familiar, which he can compare or use in order to facilitate understanding. He may want to refer to himself or other people known by the individual at risk when attempting to explain a prop's use. He needs to gently guide the individual, providing a set of written instructions showing how that prop is beneficial to him. This is, after all, a king size selling job. It is marketing at its finest!

Back to the case of the pear and the angel. By this point in the film our angel is interacting with the physician. She can now see him. He asks her to describe what a pear is like. She responds by saying the pear is sweet, juicy, soft on the tongue yet grainy like sand. The angel listens intently, but is he able to understand a pear from that description? Not really. For the angel, the pear might just as well be made of wood. For those we seek to help, lack of experiential understanding of a prop might make it as meaningless as that same pear made of wood. That being the case, it would then be our task to bring meaning to that prop by bringing relevant, previously experienced similar props into this new situation, thus providing appropriate shared and expanded understanding and meaning to that prop. That is what we mean by using previously understood props to help explain new ones.

It was said long ago, by one far greater than us, that "All the world is a stage and we are but actors." And, if this is so, then what we do now has been done for eons. After all, every stage uses props. Scenes contain props. Some scenes are rich in all kinds of props. Others contain only a few. Any scene can be broken down to almost any level to make it more understandable. Understand the props and we might be able to get the individual to understand the scene. Understand the scene and he might be able to gauge his role in that scene. Find a way to help him understand his role and appropriate interaction might begin. And as successful social interactions begin, further attempts to make contact may also expand. This is a major, long-term goal, one that is possible. To move from the outside of a room looking in, to being a part of that room's interior will take time, patience and a social facilitator. Most of us are not easily moved to accept change. Whether we have functioned in the SPAIR or SWAIR model referred to in the previous chapter, change can be difficult. We tend to prefer, even crave, a kind of sameness, often fearing or resenting the continuous change that seems to assault us, bombard us throughout life. Changes in schedule, location, event, or even a change in style, fabric or color of clothing can often result in anxiety, resentment, perhaps even feeling out of control. This is because sameness is dependable. We can count on it, lean on it. Sameness allows us to feel in control. It gives us a feeling of security. We know what to expect. We are prepared. We are confident we know how to respond because we are comfortable in our sameness, comfortable because we know what will come next.

Are those individuals at risk, those we aim this manual towards, really all that different from the rest of us? Might their need for sameness be just a matter of degree? Or is it more? Is their reluctance to accept change merely a more exaggerated form of what we need? Is it magnified by a slower rate of processing information? To take it one step farther, is it possible that the slower the rate of the processing of information, the greater the potential emotional inability to cope with what that information means?

Consider the behavioral fallout we frequently encounter when the expectations of the special needs individual do not mesh with the scene in which that individual finds himself. Say you are in an ice cream parlor. The special needs youngster has decided he wants a chocolate chip ice cream cone. But, today there is no chocolate chip ice cream. The chocolate chip ice cream truck had a breakdown this morning before dawn and all the chocolate chip ice cream on the truck has melted. The youngster has his mind set on chocolate chip. Nothing else will do; not cookies and cream, not marble fudge, not chocolate chunk! What are you going to do? How are you going to get the child to understand that there are other ice cream trucks, other ice cream parlors and stores, other ways to get the desired results? How are you going to get the individual to accept an alternate approach to the ice cream problem?

This may sound like a scenario out of the blue; yet, I am sure you might agree that situations similar to this one are not unfamiliar. In chapter eleven we will talk about the quick script form of SF, how it works and how it can be applied to the scenario we have just presented. The breakdown of SPAIR can be prevented here as in other situations by the use of SF so that an acceptable, comfortable approach to the problem helps to resolve it, bringing it to a successful, positive conclusion. In chapter eleven we will also talk about the specific form of SF we would use when out and about with your youngster, or client, at risk.

Remember the childhood story of Dumbo? Remember the feather Dumbo carried, the one he believed was necessary for him to fly? We know this feather did not create lift.

But Dumbo didn't. He needed the support this feather provided. His feather was a form of Social Facilitation, the support of something familiar, comforting and concrete.

The feather we will use will be the feather of sameness, the support of something familiar to enable risk-taking, acceptance of change and growth. In this case, we'll use props; tangible, concrete props. Why do we believe these familiar, tangible props can help?

- Because familiar, tangible props are concrete.
- Because familiar, tangible props are visual.
- Because many children with these special needs are good visual learners.
- Because something familiar is something we can count on.
- Because familiar, tangible props can give us the emotional security to gain access to desired, unfamiliar props.
- Because familiar, tangible props can provide us a base for social interchange.
- Because something familiar has comfort value.
- Because something familiar can be used to reduce possible anxiety in a new situation.
- Because something familiar can facilitate a new understanding of some previously misunderstood situation.
- Because a familiar prop can be useful in generalizing from the specific.

In essence, the prop, SF, becomes the bridge between the "SPAIR" model of the typical individual to the SWAIR model of the individual with special needs. By putting the individual back on the track to appropriate behavior so that his analysis and response is socially acceptable we are better enabling him to cope, to reach out into a frustrating and confusing world and establish a stronger foothold in it.

In the chapters that follow we will provide this foothold for you to grasp and use. We will demonstrate how to take something familiar, something tangible, something comforting and comfortable and begin to break down that something into simpler and simpler, smaller and smaller, less and less complicated units. You will learn how to keep breaking down these units until you reach something you could categorize as the smallest, simplest, least complicated, most familiar, tangible unit you need in order to help the individual at risk.

The prop, broken down to its smallest, simplest, least complicated, most familiar unit will be the foundation from which to build. It will be the starting point in establishing a baseline of communication and understanding between the individual at risk and the scenario in which that individual needs assistance. Remember, the beginning is anyplace you decide. You need only a secure, mutually familiar foundation from which to build.

Chapter VI

The Two Way Street versus the One Way Street

The Two Way Street

David can see the park from his bedroom window. Each Tuesday morning he and his mother walk across the big noisy street and into the park. The weather this Tuesday morning is particularly lovely. The birds chant their individual melodies as a soft breeze blows through the many trees that grow in the park. It is a lovely spring day.

David's mother enjoys taking him to the park. They hold hands as they cross the busy street and march toward the enormous sandbox in the park's center. The sandbox is chock full of the latest equipment, a tempting choice for any youngster. "Do you want to go on the swings or play in the sand?" she asks him.

"I want to play in the sand. May I have my sand toys?" David asks as he looks up at his Mother.

"Certainly," she says as she holds out his basket full of well-used sand implements.

As David runs off to join a group of other children already at play in the sand, his mother will sit down on a nearby bench to read a bit, a ritual which occurs each week. As she reads she will glance up, now and again, to see what David is doing. She enjoys these special moments with her son. All too soon he will be entering Kindergarten and their weekly Tuesday outings will end.

This morning there are three children at the far end of the sandbox. They are digging a giant hole in the sand. Busily they dig, construct and create. There are toy implements strewn about everywhere. There are the usual shovels, sifters and buckets, along with household plastic bowls, cups and spoons. This week's toy assortment even seems to include a few toy trucks and bulldozers.

David, arms full of toys, runs across the sandbox. He stops just short of the group. "Hi," he says, gazing at the members of the group. "I'm David. Can I play?"

The three children stop digging and look up. Spotting the toys he carries in his arms as well as his self-introduction they quickly respond. “Okay,” says one little boy directly across the gaping hole in the sand. A second child pipes up, “That’s a neat dump truck. Can I see it?” he asks. “Watch out for my castle,” says the only little girl in the group. “The princess is inside.”

David holds out the dump truck and the second youngster takes hold of it. He then sits down carefully between two children, his introduction and acceptance to the group now complete.

David’s mother glances up from her book, noting David’s newfound friends. She knows he will be busily occupied for the next hour. She smiles and resumes her reading.

The One Way Street

Brian can see the park from his bedroom window. Each Tuesday morning he and his mother walk across the big noisy street and into the park. The weather this Tuesday morning is particularly lovely. The birds chant their individual melodies as a soft breeze blows through the many trees that grow in the park. It is a lovely spring day.

Though Brian’s mother enjoys taking him to the park, she knows that she will need to keep an eye on him at all times. She holds his hand firmly as they cross the busy street and march toward the enormous sandbox in the park’s center. The sandbox is chock full of the latest equipment, a tempting choice for any youngster. “Do you want to go on the swings or play in the sand?” she asks him.

There is no reply; however, his pulling on her arm alerts her to the children playing at the far end of the sandbox and leads her to believe that is where Brian wants to go.

“Do you want to play with the children?” she asks as she looks down at the top of his head.

He continues to pull on her arm, trying to break free. “Sand,” he says. He slips his hand out from his mother’s hold and runs headlong toward an area where three youngsters are already engaged in play.

"What about your sand toys?" his mother calls out after him, holding up his basket full of well-used sand implements. Seeming not to hear nor understand or perhaps unable to stop his forward motion, Brian does not turn around, but continues running.

Unaware of the rapidly approaching Brian, the three children at the far end of the sandbox are busily digging a giant hole. They dig, construct and create. There are toy implements strewn everywhere. There are the usual shovels, sifters and buckets, along with household plastic bowls, cups and spoons. This week's toy assortment even seems to include a few toy trucks and bulldozers.

Brian's mother quickly follows him across the sandbox, wary of what might ensue, yet hoping against hope that Brian's enthusiasm and probable attempt at group play will be successful or at least somewhat acceptable. She tries to stay a safe distance away as she watches and holds her breath. Oh how she wishes these moments could be somehow different, somehow better. All too soon he will be entering Kindergarten and their weekly Tuesday sandbox journeys will end, with Brian having never successfully been able to make himself part of a group activity, even with her help.

Brian stops just before the giant hole the youngsters have dug. The three children stop digging and look up. Without a moment's hesitation Brian jumps into the hole. Tripping over the little girl's castle he sits down directly in the center of the hole. Not uttering a word he picks up a nearby shovel and begins to dig around himself.

The little girl begins to cry. "You squashed my princess," she wails.

Surprised by Brian's abrupt entry into their group the second child says, "You can't sit there. That's our giant hole. You need to get up."

Brian does not respond but continues to dig. The third child takes hold of Brian's hand and tries to pull him up and out of the hole, but finds Brian firmly entrenched.

Brian's mother quickly moves forward and takes him out of the hole. "You mustn't sit there sweetheart," she says, sitting him between the two boys. The two boys look at Brian and then at his mother.

"Why did he sit in our hole?" asks one youngster as he looks up at Brian's mother.

"He doesn't understand," she answers softly.

The youngster looks intently at Brian. He then looks back at Brian's mother. "Why doesn't he understand?" he persists.

"He's a little bit different," replies the mother.

"Oh," says the youngster. A moment later the youngster looks at Brian and asks, "What's your name?" When there is no reply he asks a second time. When Brian still says nothing the youngster points and volunteers, "I'm Justin and that's Jimmy and she's Mary."

Brian takes note of the little girl's wailing. He puts his hands up to his ears and begins to rock. His mother begins to help the little girl rebuild her castle, instantly shutting off her tears. The two young boys continue to try to interact with Brian.

"Do you want to play with us?" they ask him softly, somehow understanding, knowing that Brian is not exactly like them.

"You want to play," Brian finally responds, as he removes his hands from his ears.

Justin now hands Brian a shovel and shows him how to remove sand from the hole.

Brian shovels three or four times and then gets up and wanders off, never looking back. Brian's mother smiles and thanks the children. She then heads off after her son.

End of engagement!

Unlike young David in the "Two Way Street" example, children with some kind of Pervasive Developmental Disorder, children like Brian who are developmentally different, may not take internal cues and use them to interact with others. However, others may approach and initiate social contact. Using the example of the sandbox, the special needs child will either stay on the perimeter or utilize props in a vacuum, that is, as if no other people were present. Other children will approach in a social fashion and initiate. Hence, the one-way street.

This concept, though unexplored, can be extrapolated to other situations. Is it possible that the pronoun reversal ("You want to play" instead of "I want to play"), once thought to be merely a reversal of speech, MAY, in fact, be a manifestation of this "One way street"? By relying on the "you" rather than the "I" in a statement, the special needs child is utilizing external (another person's) cues to fulfill his or her own needs. Things from the outside are brought inside with little going the other way. The all too familiar "you" may indicate more than just an error in noun use but refer to the greater form of me. He doesn't have internal cues. Therefore, he relies on the external which he then incorporates within, as his own. And because the special needs child has difficulty "producing" on his own relative to social interactions, he often latches onto others, other's belongings, etc. as his own. He does this to "nourish" this need. Hence, the "you" may be a manifestation of this need and subsequent gratification.

For example, I heard a story one day, supposedly true, concerning a unique individual in his late twenties. It seems that his parents were giving a large dinner party for some friends. Just as the group was about to sit down to dinner out comes the young man stark naked into the dining room. "Tell me to turn off the shower," he said to his mother. She quickly obliged and he turned around and walked off. It was not that he was unwilling to turn off the shower by himself. He was either unable to do it or never considered doing it. His mother was connected to the process. He had to pull her in to complete the task.

By utilizing Social Facilitation "SF" we can design a targeted story or group of stories that will lay the foundation for Brian's better understanding of his sandbox experience.

Social Facilitation is a means of taking a child who only understands or is most comfortable on a one-way street and gently guiding him down the two way street. In this fashion the child or adult can better adapt to life's highways.

To meet our goal of finding a way to enable Brian to not stay on the perimeter of the group or run off after a short time, but rather to be able to integrate into the social circle and respond more like David, we need to use Social Facilitation techniques to design an appropriate tool to help Brian successfully meet his needs. The work we do in the pages ahead will try to meet this goal. The work we do together can begin to take the individual with special needs from his world of the one way street into the world of the two way street.

Chapter VII

Mine versus Yours / Sameness versus Change

Let us conduct a small experiment. Take a pencil and paper. Observe and write down how you perceive that your youngster responds in word and action to the various rooms in his home. Begin with his or her room, followed by your room. Next, observe his or her response to rooms in another home, perhaps the home of a close friend or relative. Remember to keep in mind his familiarity with the other homes you choose to use. Then answer these questions for yourself:

- How calm does he or she appear in the other home versus his?
- Is there any hesitancy to enter one room more than another? If so, which ones?
- Does he appear restless, stiff, or anxious to enter or leave?
- Is he pacing, shouting, using other odd, repetitive behaviors, or showing other signs of discomfort?
- How does he respond to a visit to a model home?

Rank the differences in his or her behavior when placed in each of these places. After you have ranked the various homes from the most comforting to the least, begin to think about how each of these surroundings differ from his home.

Your goal will be to try and learn where, when, why and how his behaviors vary. If you can begin to understand his reactions, those reactions can be cited in a story. In this way you can help him help himself. As he begins to understand what behaviors are appropriate in what environments and why, he can begin to develop a framework from which he can move forward. Oftentimes an individual may pace back and forth, unable to proceed, because he is uncertain about what he is supposed to do. He is unable to consciously find a solution to his dilemma and perhaps even to clearly recognize it, but merely feels a generalized anxiety. It is our job to help this individual recognize and consciously define a problem situation and then take it to the next step, that of verbally expressing his concern. In some ways our observing their difficulty and helping define that problem for them both in picture and written form is the method to broach and breech the problem.

When we are able to do this, we will be able to help the individual respond to the new surroundings, in terms of feelings and in terms of anxiety, as well as he or she does to the home environment. How can this be achieved? It can be achieved in many ways.

Though the individual in need may be your client and not your child, let us proceed as if this situation were to begin in your home and this were your child.

Take a camera and photograph your bedroom and your child's bedroom. Take photos when each room is tidy and when each room is messy.

When the photos are developed, group them by room. How you present the material depends on the age and level of the individual. Remember, you are concretely presenting information in visual form, which the person probably knows on some other level. We are going to go from the seemingly simple to the more complex.

Here's the beginning of a story or album.

This is my room.
Sometimes my room is tidy.
When my room is tidy my bed is made.
When my room is tidy my toys are put away.
When my room is tidy my clothes are put away.

I like my room.
Being in my room makes me feel good.

[leave sufficient space between paragraphs and place a snapshot of the tidy room here]

Sometimes my room is not tidy.
Sometimes my room is messy.
My room is messy when my bed is not made.
My room is messy when my toys are not put away.
I like my room even when it is messy.
Being in my room makes me feel good.

[leave sufficient space between paragraphs and place a snapshot of the messy room here]

This is my Mom's room.
Sometimes my Mom's room is tidy.
When my Mom's room is tidy her bed is made.
When my Mom's room is tidy her clothes are put away.
My Mom likes her room.
Being in her room makes my Mom feel good.

[leave sufficient space between paragraphs and place a snapshot of Mom's tidy room here]

Sometimes my Mom's room is not tidy.
Sometimes my Mom's bed is not made.
Sometimes my Mom's clothes are not put away.
My Mom likes her room even when it is messy.
Being in her room makes my Mom feel good.

[leave sufficient space and place a snapshot of Mom's messy room here]

This is not a story about keeping a bedroom tidy and neat. Nor is it a story about defining what is yours and what is mine or learning the appropriate skills to enable an individual to gain access to something that belongs to another. This story is even more basic. This is a story to demonstrate the fact that there *are* things known as yours and other things that are not yours and are known as mine. This is a story to demonstrate that we each have things that are within our own personal domain and that we may have special feelings associated with these things. Mother has things. They are in her domain. She may have special feelings that I don't have which are associated with those things. This is a story to demonstrate, in a simple way, a fairly complex set of circumstances whereby we begin to recognize what is ours versus what is not. We may begin to understand that what is ours is different from what is our Mom's.

The story could go on to talk about what belongs to my relative or friend versus what is mine. We could then go on to talk about kinds of feelings and behaviors that are appropriate toward each. Once we understand the comfort of our own rooms in our house, we could move on to the home of another.

Pick a relative's home. Take the same type of pictures over a few days. Point out to your child that these rooms, both tidy and messy, belong to other people (whoever those other people are) and that these people like their rooms just as you and your youngster like your rooms.

You can take the same information and take photos of a friend's home. If you feel uncomfortable using a bedroom, use a kitchen, family room or dining room. Take photos with your child's age mate in their room and your neighbor in her dining room or kitchen. Take lots and lots of photos.

Almost like a geometry problem, the material can be broken down, in fact, must be broken down, to logical discrete units. Note the following example:

This is not my home.
This is Johnny's home.
Johnny's house is not my house.
Johnny likes his house.

Our houses are different.
And that is okay.

[leave sufficient space between paragraphs and place a snapshot of Johnny and his house here]

Johnny is my friend.
Johnny has his own bedroom.
This is Johnny's room.
Johnny likes his room.
Johnny's room looks different from my room.
This is because Johnny is different from me.
We are different and our rooms are different.
And that is okay.

[leave sufficient space between paragraphs and place a snapshot of Johnny in his room here]

This is Johnny's Mom's room.
Johnny's Mom's room belongs to her.
I may not go into her room unless I am invited.
My Mom may not go into Johnny's Mom's room unless she is invited.

[leave sufficient space and place a snapshot of Johnny's Mom's room here]

You can continue this story, going through other portions of the house and yard. On and on, as much as is needed or, at least, as much as you have time to write. Note that one story does not need to capture it all. Stories can be short or long, depending on need, difficulty of material and the time necessary to create them and, of course, the level of the individual in need.

What is important to remember is that when we write we refrain from becoming judgmental. Much of what we write should be descriptive. It can include idiomatic expressions and what those expressions mean. It should answer the how and the why of a situation, providing useful solutions. The story can go in any direction you deem necessary. If the concept of yours versus mine is still not concrete enough you could break it down further by, perhaps, providing stickers saying “mine,” “not mine,” “Johnny’s,” “Mom’s,” etc. In this concrete “how to” way, the individual could, hands on, have a way to see the difference. It provides him with another tool for understanding.

For those individuals who have difficulty identifying an appropriate internal emotion toward a particular situation, inserting a few words associated with an emotion can be useful in helping identify that feeling. For example, in chapter four we talked about the boy and the neighbor’s new computer. We talked about the boy’s bewilderment at the neighbor’s response to him. In an SF story we could talk about his excitement and how computers make him feel happy. At the same time we would give him a few directive sentences, sentences to tell him what to do. Most importantly, as author Carol Gray points out in her wonderful books, the use of statements directing the reader to carry out or refrain from certain behaviors should be used less frequently than descriptive ones. In this case, the directive sentences would tell him that he would need to wait until the following day before he could go over to the neighbor’s house. He would have to wait until a specific time before he could go next door and ask permission to see or use the computer. Further, he would have to understand that just because he asks to see or use that computer does not mean the neighbor’s response will be yes. Sometimes the answer will be no. SF would help him to learn to cope with that potential “no” response.

We want the reader to enjoy all the tools of Social Facilitation and use them as needed. We want him to think of them like a thirsty man thinks about a glass of water; that he needs them, can have access to them, and can use them any time the need arises.

Chapter VIII

The Lunch Group

I was having lunch with four friends, all mothers of children with some form of autism, Asperger's Syndrome or other developmental difficulty. We meet weekly and spend most of our time discussing issues regarding our children. One woman has two sons, one who, she says, is clearly autistic; the other she believes to now fall under the newer Asperger Syndrome definition. I say that because at four years old this child did not speak and at five still had many self-stimulatory behaviors characteristic of autism itself. The balance of the lunch group have children who either fall under the traditional Kanner definition most of us know to be autism or some other developmental disability.

Something had been on my mind and so I decided to pose a question to the group this particular day. "Do your children expect you to know the answers to all questions?" I asked. Each sat a moment and thought about my question. One by one they each nodded their head. "Yes," they agreed unanimously. No matter how high-functioning, no matter what the school placement or age of child, no matter what the diagnosis to date, every child had to have their parent be the concrete pillar of knowledge on any topic as well as be the master of any problem's resolution. Perhaps this is true of most young children. However, in this case there is a refusal or inability to understand or accept any explanation to the contrary. In addition, this unshakable belief can go on for years.

"How does your youngster respond if you tell him you don't know the answer to his question? How does he respond if you tell him you cannot fix something?" I asked. "Give me an example."

The first mother begins. Her son is not quite fourteen years old, fairly verbal and often echolalic. "When Alan (not his real name) was four or five, he would bring me his broken toy and demand that I fix it."

"What happened if the toy was not fixable?" I asked.

"That was not an option," replied the mother. "It HAD to be fixed. If it couldn't, he couldn't handle it. He would become severely agitated."

"How did you resolve the problem?" I queried.

"I don't know. I just kept trying to show him and tell him that this toy couldn't be fixed," she replied.

"Then what?" I pursued.

"Well," she said, "he would tantrum for quite a while. He'd be banging on doors with his fists and kicking with his feet. It was not a pretty picture."

"How did it end?" I asked.

"I usually promised to buy him a new toy if he would quiet down."

"Does he still insist you be able to fix a toy or replace it; or can he accept the fact that some things are neither fixable nor replaceable?" I asked.

She thought for a moment. "No, he still has a hard time," she replied honestly. "I just can't seem to get him to understand. But, I can bargain a little more with him now that he is older. I tell him we can get a new one for his next birthday. He has a birthday list in his room."

I can just imagine how large that list is!

The second mother told a variation of that story. Her son, diagnosed as having Asperger's Syndrome only a year or two ago and now eighteen years old and out of high school, had spent the day working for a general contractor. The contractor, she said, liked her son and his work. He told her son to call him the following Monday morning if he felt he would like to work. The contractor was busy and could use the help.

Come Monday morning, her son didn't make the call. Instead he sat by the telephone waiting. "Why didn't you call the contractor?" his mother later asked. "Didn't you like the work?"

"Yes," answered her son. "But he should have called me. He should have known I wanted to work."

Needless to say his mother was dumbfounded.

A third mother decided to speak. Her son seemed to get most of his interpretations off the movie screen or television, she told the rest of the group. He did not seem to be able to express any clear, unique understanding of things separate from what he viewed on the television or movie screen. He appeared to have no views of his own. Instead, who he was and what he perceived was dependent upon what he garnered from the outside world and brought into himself.

It was apparent that no matter how high functioning our kids, no matter how mild or severe, no matter what the variation in diagnosis, each of them had, in one form or another, a similar difficulty. The other person had to know what was in their mind or put something in their mind. The other person had to be able to know, to do, to fix, to solve riddles and problems without being asked or consulted. The other was the keeper of all knowledge and responsible for all solutions. The stimulus had to come from the outside.

Indeed, that even appears in the way many of these children learn to speak. It often seems as if the way in which they use their mother tongue is like you and I learning a foreign language, taking words and phrases and plugging them in. It is a conscious and constant effort. How many of us spoke to the developmentally different youngster and got an echolalic response? "You want a cookie?" we'd ask. And the response would be, "You want a cookie," meaning "I want a cookie." We referred to them as "you", so they responded to themselves as "you". They took the question and turned it into a response, thus trying to interact with you and get what they desired.

Is their language related to an inability to separate who they are from the rest of the world? Is their use of language the key to understanding where their deficits lie? Perhaps it is not just semantics and the need for speech therapy that should guide our footsteps in helping these individuals. Perhaps it is their entire persona that is linked to their verbal expressive qualities. "You want a cookie," with the identical response may demonstrate this inability to separate you from me, themselves from other.

Why can't we seem to break through the impasse, which enables these individuals to realize that others are just that, O T H E R? Other, not same! Separate, not part of! How can we get them to understand that others have flaws and doubts, different flaws and doubts than they have? How can we get them to understand that others make mistakes, that mistakes they make are theirs alone, and that mistakes are both acceptable and a part of life?

Take a traditional classroom setting. A teacher asks her class to watch a certain television program one evening. The next day she breaks up the class into groups of four or five. "What was the program about?" she asks. "What did you learn?"

If you and I could listen in on the conversation of each group, what would we hear? Would the kids all say the same things? Highly unlikely! More likely, each child might have focused upon different things in the program. Certainly there would have been certain similarities, and overall the understanding of what the show was about might be similar. Yet, each child would most certainly have a slightly different perspective of the event. That perspective is guided by that child's background, experience, family structure, genetics, perceived peer pressure to express oneself honestly, etc.

In addition, as the group discussed their individual interpretations there might begin to develop a kind of appreciation of one another's perspectives. Some people might begin to see the show in a whole new light, incorporating new ideas into their own internal understanding. "I never thought of that," one might say. Assertiveness, aggressiveness, would play themselves out and ultimately a group consensus might begin to form.

Though each individual had the potential to contribute something of value to the discussion there may have been one youngster who insisted his or her point of view was the "correct" one. He or she may have had to defend that position with "proof," if not by other, more childlike means. "Oh, yeah, prove it!" says one youngster. Children begin to learn the art of persuasion, defending a position, a point of view. Leaving aggression, as a possible form of persuasion, out of the picture for a moment, look at all the shared learning that is going on. More than that, note that each person has some type of individual, internal perspective that he knows is his. He knows that Johnny's opinion is not necessarily what he has in his mind. He knows that Amy's opinions do not necessarily match Johnny's or his own. Each of them has a perspective unique to himself or herself, and separate from the other.

Individuals will share perspectives and defend positions. They garner support from the rest of the group hoping to suppress minority views. They try to establish a united interpretation through group means.

What about group perspectives? When this same teacher asks the groups to present their interpretations of the television program, would each group's version be identical? Hardly! Each group would, most likely, view certain areas in the same light, but there could be distinct variations between them.

In order for there to be one perspective for the entire class, the same process which was used for the smaller groups would once again come into play with the class as a whole. There would be give and take, each conflicting view complicating the playing field. There would be group persuasion and pressure. And finally, some overall consensus would, hopefully, ensue.

Wouldn't it be wonderful if children with developmental difficulties could begin to take part in this process? Wouldn't it be wonderful for them to witness the give and take, the varying ideas and views? Wouldn't it be wonderful if they could begin to appreciate the smorgasbord of ideas that could spring forth from each of the peers in such a group setting? Wouldn't it be wonderful if we could introduce the possibility of variation in interpretation; and that variation in interpretation is healthy? Wouldn't it be wonderful if we could get across the idea that each person can see things uniquely? And most importantly, wouldn't it be wonderful if, after exposure to various interpretations, these individuals could then decide what perspective is most comforting and comfortable to them?

This area of development is crucial for those with developmental disabilities to begin to understand. And through the Social Facilitation techniques we shall be using, even these tough, tough areas can be addressed and modified, which is where the written format comes into play.

Consider our own responses to the visual format. How often do we doubt the written word? Until, perhaps, the last few years, many of us believed almost anything we read in print. What appeared in written form was etched in stone. If it was written, it had to be true!

Not so about what we hear. You and I measure, evaluate and oftentimes discard or quickly forget what we hear. Often we don't even really hear the words as spoken. Perhaps we don't even process them. Because we are unable to see the spoken word it can disappear as the breeze passing your cheek on a hot summer day. For many individuals at risk the oral word presents this same difficulty, whereas the written format may not.

When an individual with autism, Asperger's Syndrome, or some other form of developmental difficulty is exposed to some form of Social Facilitation he can take his time analyzing a situation. We can make the writing as simple and one-sided as we like. We can also expand it. We can play the same game the teacher used above when she asked her class to break into groups and evaluate a television program. We can visually interpret the same data from more than one perspective. We can show that differing opinions are valuable and acceptable. We can even point out that mistakes can be vital to the learning process, a good thing. We can give the individual at risk as much variation as he or she can handle. And we can do it with a smile.

Perhaps, in the beginning, we might choose to provide only one perspective, our own, with more involved perspectives and variations coming in a later piece. Even if we are providing the individual with our own unique understanding of a situation, we are, nonetheless, providing him with a worldview, even if it is temporarily limited. Think of the young man with Asperger's Syndrome who sat by the telephone all day waiting for the employer to call him instead of making the call himself. If this young man understood his role to secure the job for another day or week, if he understood what he had to do and why, he might have been happily working instead of sitting at home by the telephone.

The discussion we had that day, like so many other days, was quite useful. We each came away with new insight about our kids and others like them.

Chapter IX

Social Facilitation In Action

You've been jolted into consciousness during the night by the deep rumble of an earthquake accompanied by the sounds of shattering glass and frenetic movement. Having been thrown from your bed, you grope your way toward the door jam, desperately trying to find your balance. The smell of danger, the touch of destiny, the fear generated by a world gone topsy-turvy, shakes you to your very soul. Faced with a situation in which you have not one shred of control, no way to make it stop, you hold on with every ounce of strength at your disposal and wait, wondering when your world will reestablish order.

Within a few seconds or minutes the deep rumbling sounds begin to subside, the movements slow, and your sense of balance returns. The world seems to have been restored. You have survived.

But dare you move? If so, where? How? On all fours? On two feet? And where are your slippers? Are they where you last placed them? What about your flashlight? The world is totally black; no light anywhere. You strain to hear. You know who you are, but not exactly where you are. You know where you were. But is that reality still valid? Are the parameters of the world the same? If you move in this world of darkness without benefit of slippers or flashlight, will you remain safe? Is your world the same as you last remember it? Or, has it changed? If so, how?

Groping for the light switch, you discover it does not work. You are left in total blackness, hearing only the sounds of dogs barking and the squeaks of chandeliers still swinging wildly about. You reach under the bed for a flashlight, a radio, something to connect you with reality, community.

Do we dare compare the chaos of a world erupting, changing, and crumbling from an earthquake with the world of a human trapped in the mystifying world of the developmentally disabled?

If we can equate the two and if that was the world we perceived each day, wouldn't we feel isolated, anxiety-ridden, disconnected and alone? Wouldn't we crave a return to what we had previously understood as the parameters of our world? If our world were to pose a constant threat to us through unexpected, unwanted change, isn't is possible that we could feel like we were trapped in an ongoing earthquake? Might it not also be true that the more significantly afflicted one is by these kinds of disabilities, the more unstable and frightening the world might be? If this is so, is it any wonder that these individuals often respond as they do; overwhelmed, bombarded, out of control?

What if we not only found ourselves in darkness, but were also being bombarded by sound, visual stimuli, sickening smells and harsh touch? What if our world were filled with pain and confusion? And what if no one understood?

Where would we go? Where would we hide? To children with Autism, Asperger's Syndrome, Pervasive Developmental Disorders, and other developmental difficulties, few of the props and characters surrounding them on a daily basis are well understood. Not only do subtle cues and innuendoes remain unseen or misunderstood, but even more major moves, situational shifts and concepts often remain a mystery as well. The anxiety, uncertainty and fear created can become overwhelming and debilitating. They can result in the negative, inappropriate, maladaptive behaviors we sometimes see.

Surely a chair is concrete, stationary and dependable. It remains motionless. Humanity is, on the other hand, a source of constant motion. Live things move leaving the individual at risk in a perpetual state of anxiety. He cannot maintain his balance because he cannot fathom you in motion. He is vulnerable and threatened by a world of motion, a world of confusion, a world he cannot pin down or label, a fluid world of change.

Perhaps we should look at it another way. Have you ever taken part in a group function that was intended to make you feel like you were slow, had learning disabilities, or were just plain different from others? If you have, you know how many aspirin it took to get rid of the headache you felt that day. If you haven't, consider yourself just plain lucky!

A few years back ten of us were "privileged" to be part of such a group. What transpired that day can only be expressed as an experiment in torture. For three miserable hours we suffered through a first class emotional bruising, pummeled by an instructor, skilled in the art of making the participant feel inadequate.

If, in that short amount of time, our self-esteem could be shattered, literally decimated, if our self-worth could be obliterated in one morning session, how do children who may inadvertently be exposed to such instruction each day emotionally survive? Where do they get the strength to return each day, knowing that they don't fit, that they're different, that no matter how hard they try many things remain beyond their grasp?

There are not enough Band-Aids to cover the wounds left by years of being on the outside. No matter how many medications or behavioral techniques we develop to help these individuals, some still just don't fit.

Yet, it's our job to help them fit. It's our job to bridge the gap between the individual's social/emotional understanding and the demands of the situation. It's our job to be that conduit for these individuals so that they are able to feel more successful, more socially, intellectually, and behaviorally integrated with society at large.

That's what Social Facilitation is all about! It seeks to fill a gap. It seeks to fill a need. "SF", as we call it, is a customized and individualized tool to broaden understanding. It is a tool to widen the limited field of vision and understanding so that a more panoramic view can be seen and understood. Social Facilitation is an approach designed to help the individual at risk so that he or she will be better able to respond in a more socially acceptable manner.

Picture yourself an actor in a motion picture. In your hand you hold a script. This script includes several scenes in which you have a role to play. Having read the script in its entirety, you not only have a fair understanding of your role and character, you probably have a fair understanding of other characters in the script as well. Beyond the other characters, you somehow understand the need for and use of the various props and costumes to be used throughout the movie.

But what if you had no script? What if you had no understanding of your character or any other character? What if the various props and costumes to be used were a complete mystery to you? What if you had no idea how one character related to another? What if you even had some difficulty relating by language and even by gesture? What then?

Take Joe, for example. Joe who? Just an actor named Joe. Let's assume that Joe is a normal kind of Joe. Joe is, for want of a better word, an "NT," a neurotypical sort of guy, a "normie". Without benefit of script or any foreknowledge, we dump this poor fellow into a scene on the planet Neptune. We tell him, "Joe, you're on the planet Neptune." But that's all we tell him.

Being a "normie", our Joe isn't exactly thrilled at the predicament in which we have placed him. He would like to complain but holds his tongue. After all, this is his big chance in the movies. He takes a few deep breaths and makes mental note of the fact that he has no adequate tools to play this role as he surmises it should be played. Without benefit of script he knows he will not have a clear understanding of his surroundings, as well as issues of safety. Yet, somehow he begins to piece it together by drawing on his past. Having suffered through a basic astronomy course in his college days, Joe quickly tries to recall everything, anything about the planet Neptune. Though this doesn't yield a whole lot of information, he finally comes up with one fact. Neptune is far from the sun.

Let's add another ingredient to the mix. We'll sprinkle a time constraint, an additional stressor, into our mix. Since time is money and our producer needs to make the most of his limited funding, shooting will start immediately.

Act one. Scene one.

We place Joe in a fake rocket ship, our Neptunian Express. "Your hibernation chamber has opened early due to a fire," we tell him. "You'll need to abandon ship."

Adrenaline pumping like crazy, Joe looks around. He sees the Halloween quality spacesuit we've provided, some freeze-dried space food and his blaster (that's all we could afford). We remind him that he's to leave the Neptunian Express immediately.

"Action!" the director calls out.

"What action?" Joe's mind is going a mile a minute. Anxiety? By the carload! However, within a short time, Joe takes a deep breath and settles down, allowing himself to engage in a bit of rational thinking.

Neptune is far from the sun, he reminds himself, as his mind musters up other bits of "Astronomy One" data. It's probably quite chilly out there. Neptune's distance from the sun probably means there is little sunlight. Neptune is a gas giant. Can the surface support me? He wonders for a moment until he realizes the surface is already supporting the Neptunian Express. But what about the availability of oxygen? What about gravity? What about wind? What about other possible unknown dangers?

"Time's a fleeting Joe," says the director.

"Wait! Wait!" pleads Joe, sweat now visible on his brow.

"No time, Joe," says the director. "Act one. Scene one."

Joe turns his head. His eyes focus on his spacesuit hanging on a hook. Having seen pictures of astronauts wearing spacesuits in documentaries, he quickly begins to put it on. But, putting it on seems to be no easy feat. The suit is heavy, even by Neptunian standards, whatever those are; and the fasteners are a bit unusual. He has no time to lose. The chamber is fast filling with smoke. But, he just can't seem to get the darn fasteners to close. Spying some tape on a nearby counter he resorts to taping himself closed. "There!" he says to himself. "Finally!"

Lights! Camera! Action (again)! The smoke thickens (and so does the plot). With much trepidation and a wildly beating heart Joe opens the hatch and begins to descend an unstable aluminum ladder, beginning to doubt his abilities and wishing he had never agreed to take part in this endeavor. The hard cloak containing his self-esteem is beginning to crack. He desperately wants to bolt!

"Concentrate Joe," shouts the director who senses Joe's distress. "Get ahold of yourself."

Joe takes another deep breath. Okay, he says to himself. You can do this! Or can you? Joe's earlier internal questions continue to haunt him. Air? Gravity? Never mind air and gravity!

What in the world, he says out loud, as his eyes feast upon the wildest, weirdest-looking creatures he could ever have imagined. In the midst of all Joe's confusion and terror he suddenly finds himself being greeted by rather large amoebae-like, green, featureless creatures that appear to enjoy rubbing their bodies on thorny, blinking, scraggly, smelly, plantlike structures. The creatures hobble on over. They soon surround Joe, splashing green goo on his helmet as they gurgle and hiss. Are they being aggressive? Is this their way of saying "Hello"? Is this a kind of rollicking-frolicking play? Or is he to be dinner?

Joe is the only earthling among the many strange green-goo givers. Their behavior is totally bewildering to him. Is he going to "freak-out?" Is he going to collapse into a jelly-like blob of flesh amidst goo? What is he supposed to do? How is he going to play this role? Indeed, how could he play his role?

How much easier this role would have been had Joe been given a script, a pictorial representation of the fantasy world in which he was to play a role. How much less anxiety and fear Joe would have suffered had he been offered some functional, concrete framework from which to embark. But, alas, Joe was given no such script, no such framework.

We'll come back to this seemingly absurd scenario toward the close of the chapter. Joe's a good guy. He'll hold it together. The question is, is this scenario as far-fetched as it seems? If you and I had been diagnosed with some form of autism, Asperger's Syndrome, or some other developmental disability, how would we fare on the Neptunian Express? How would we fare when presented with new and seemingly foreign scenes, scenes for which we were not privy to all the tools we would need in order to cope, in order to function adequately? Does it seem fair to say that we might respond in a similar fashion to Joe? And what if our fear and anxiety level were always on high beam, in contrast to the cool nature we have given our Joe?

Imagine another scene. Meet Johnny. Johnny sits in a classroom. We'll make it a full-inclusion class, with Johnny as its only youngster having a developmental disability. Johnny sits in the middle of the room at his desk. He is surrounded by his classmates. His teacher sits in front of the class at her desk. Johnny can see his classmates. He can see his teacher.

His desk is his safety net. It is the same "warm fuzzy" desk he occupies each day. His classroom and his desk make up part of his home away from home. Johnny has come to understand the world of his classroom, the arrangement of students, chairs, blackboard, etc. through the lens of his seat. Yet the periodic movement of his teacher, the constant movement of other students, and the shuffling of schedules keep Johnny on edge.

If a fellow classmate temporarily occupies a seat not assigned to him, Johnny's anxiety level goes up. If a group of students decide to turn their chairs to face one another for a group discussion, thus disrupting the classroom order, he becomes more upset. Johnny cannot be at ease. The pace of change is too rapid. He does not understand what his classmates do or why they are doing it. Their constant movements and interplay with one another and occasionally with him keep him in a constant state of anxiety. For him the world is often in fast-forward mode. For him, intensely focusing on something of interest helps reduce his stress and anxiety. For him, disappearing into a favorite book or a series of complex math problems helps to calm his fears.

How much easier Johnny's life might be if the favorite book in front of him could be a script, a pictorial representation of his classroom world, a world in which he played a role. How much less anxiety and fear he would have, if he had an adaptable concrete framework from which to embark. But, alas, Johnny has no such script, no such framework.

One of the youngsters throws a paper airplane at Johnny. The rest of the class laughs. The teacher looks up from her desk and tells the class to quiet down. The interchange lasted a few seconds. No matter how he tried, Johnny did not fully comprehend what had just happened. Consequently, his anxiety began to rise and he tried even harder to focus, to bury himself in the book he held in front of his face.

How different is Johnny's world from the scenario in which we have placed Joe and his green-goo throwing amoebae-like creatures?

Let's move on to a third situation. Imagine a lecture hall full of college students. The speaker is hypnotic, the listeners spellbound, rapt by his words. Midway through the lecture a young woman busily chewing bubble gum speaks out. Her question breaks the spell of the speaker's words. The speaker graciously responds. However, it is not long before the young woman, now squirming in her seat, blurts out another question, and yet another, and still another. A dialogue between speaker and student ensues, so that what initially seemed to be a single break in continuity was becoming an uncomfortable situation.

The audience, while initially polite, begins to show signs of impatience, a dull roar echoing through the hall each time another question is volleyed from the insistent young woman. Finally, the speaker suggests the young woman see him afterwards.

A calmness returns to the lecture hall. Soon, however, the young woman's voice can be heard again. Not even the mumbling and grumbling of the other attendees serves to quiet her persistent verbiage. She is seemingly oblivious.

What is wrong with this woman? Why did she break from an accepted unspoken code, a decorum which you and I know goes with attendance at such a lecture? What went wrong? Didn't she understand her role as a passive listener within a group? Didn't she understand how inappropriate her behavior was, especially after having been told what to do next? Wasn't she able to control herself? Or, is it possible that she just did not understand appropriate and acceptable behavior in this situation?

How much better the same lecture would have gone had the young woman been given a script, a pictorial representation of a lecture situation, a situation in which she played a role as a passive listener. Had she been aware of acceptable rules of conduct in this situation perhaps she would have behaved in a manner more suitable to that situation. But, alas, the young woman had no such script, no such framework from which to operate. Like Joe and Johnny she was operating at a loss.

So what am I saying? I am suggesting that for those with Autism, Asperger's Syndrome, or some other Pervasive Developmental Disorder or difficulty, the ever new and changing social situation can present potential problems and dilemmas. Like Joe and the amoebas, Johnny and his classmates and the young woman at the lecture, people with these kinds of difficulties frequently find themselves immersed in situations over which they have limited understanding and limited or no control. Subtle cues as well as major ones, cues that you and I would pick up in a moment, may be totally missed or misunderstood.

Without the means to break down situations into discrete, visual, understandable, concrete segments, many individuals become overwhelmed. Cluttered and clouded by uncertainty and anxiety their response to these situations might very well be quite negative; their frustration, fear and anxiety leading to a response many would consider inappropriate and maladaptive. But how might we respond, given the same parameters of understanding?

A key to helping Joe or Johnny and even the young woman at the lecture could lie in something as simple as visual aids, a kind of visual road map. Why visual? Because an area of great strength for many of these individuals, young and old alike, is their ability to home in on the miniscule, see the concrete, focus on visual stimuli, especially stationary visual stimuli.

Not long ago I received a letter from a young man who described himself as having Asperger's Syndrome. Within the contents of that note was his disclosure of his need to focus. "Focus is the only thing in life I'm truly interested in," he wrote. He explained his need to focus in the following way. He suggested that some people have an ability to intensely focus on visual stimuli, preferably stationary visual stimuli. Words, photographs, drawings can be a very strong suit for them, perhaps the best suit!

Suppose you had a football team of athletic autistic kids (we'll use the term "autistic" as a generic term for individuals with similar disorders, though this might offend the purists). Would that be a good thing or a disaster? It depends upon how you frame the idea. Let's explore parallel paths of neurotypical and autistic individuals leading to the same goal but meeting different needs.

In order to have a successful performance, the typical individual needs to increase his or her focus by doing four things. He needs to:

- block out both internal and external stimuli;
- increase attention;
- block out emotional reactions which may interfere with focus; and
- allow creativity not to be inhibited by conventional norms.

The unimpaired individual has the ability to understand the societal norms. Surprisingly, this can work to their detriment as an inhibitory factor. A considerable amount of time is spent by them trying to achieve these four actions. Hypnosis, which is nothing more than hyperfocusing, is often utilized. In sports endeavors individuals practice "visualization" in order to "see themselves being successful." People practice rehearsal strategies until the correct action becomes more automatic. The successful performance meets the need of the "normie" by making him a hero, star, or, obviously, a success, which is the goal.

In order to have a successful performance (not necessarily in his or her eyes, but in the eyes of the rest of the world), an individual with a more mild form of autism may take a completely different path. He might easily and frequently block out external stimuli, often much to the dismay of those around him. He may have a keen natural ability to super focus on a task or object, or in technical terms is hypervigilant. He may not have to block out emotional reactions that interfere with focus because he may not be entirely cognizant of or understand empathetic reactions. And lastly, he may have a somewhat limited understanding of conventional societal norms and, therefore, may not be bound by them. This is an asset, allowing him to "see" things the typical individual may not. One could wonder why we don't see more autistic spectrum disordered football athletes.

In order for many individuals to be successful in terms of the normie's world, they simply must rehearse the appropriate behavior. We know that many individuals with some form of autism don't need to be heroes, stars, or even successes, though certainly many do find a reward in astounding others. However, many are extremely motivated to focus on something. In fact, focusing to such depths that the world is totally washed away may be what autism is all about. It is often why a subject such as mathematics holds such intrigue for them, precise, exact and systematized. It is consistent, dependable and reliable.

Social Facilitation makes use of the visual strengths and ability to focus that are found in many of these individuals. Depth of focus is an asset. Social Facilitation works because it fits the patterns and needs of the autistic population like a key in a lock. In fact, it may unlock many of the abilities of the individual at risk, turning what are normally considered liabilities into assets.

Our ultimate goal is the same – societally defined successful performance and behavior. The neurotypical individual and the autistic one are just getting there by different paths and for different reasons.

Behavior modification focuses on acceptable behavior, not on a philosophical discussion of why the person is doing the behavior. Let's go back to our football team. Suppose members of the team were unaffected by the need to be superheroes. Suppose that the sport simply offered them a means of superfocusing on information. There would be no fear of failure, nor fear of success. They would be able to concentrate all their efforts on focusing. A running back, for example, might be able to run through a field of defenders as if he had a road map, eluding would be tacklers all the way to the goal line. Ridiculous? Not at all. Think of what coaches demand of their athletes on a regular basis–concentrate, focus, be intense, see yourself as getting to the goal. The autistic individual with athletic ability may have a distinct advantage over his neurotypical counterpart. Pity the poor sports journalist trying to do a post-game interview!

Social Facilitation is the road map to the goal line of socialization. The individual with autism may not pick up the social cues necessary to interact appropriately because those cues are often too abstract to be an object of focusing. A social script, on the other hand, is quite specific. When properly constructed, it contains all the elements necessary to guide the individual through the maze of misunderstanding and arrive at the appropriate social action, not just for the purpose of being successful in his or her mind, but also for the purpose of being able to superfocus.

As with any analysis of behavior, there remains no "generic" PDD, ADD or LD individual. Each person is an individual with unique characteristics, traits, and behaviors. Social Facilitation should be viewed as a tool in the hands of a skilled practitioner or artist and not as a panacea for autism.

As a parent, teacher, aide, nurse, physician, therapist or other interested party, let us make you the expert, so that you can be the one who can break down a scene into its basic components. You can be the one to reveal the hidden meaning behind and between characters and props. You can be the one to make the world a more comforting, comfortable place to be, revealing order from previously perceived chaos.

Putting the same information in order, Social Facilitation (SF) can help you:

1. Break down social interactions to their basic components.

2. Reveal hidden meaning behind verbal and visual interplay between characters.

3. Visually define need for specific props.

4. Show interplay between props and characters.

5. Expand social understanding between characters.

6. Broaden understanding of an entire scene.

You don't need to be a professional writer. You need only have:

- A desire to help.
- A pen and quick script pad or any pencil and pad.
- A camera and film.
- An understanding of when and how to use which type of SF.

Social Facilitation is a process by which social understanding may be enhanced through visual means. Social Facilitation involves:

1. The observation of the individual who needs help.

2. Interviews with individuals who interact with the person at risk.

3. Defining a problem.

4. A desire to change.

5. A course of action to accomplish change.

6. Determination of type of social scripting to be used.

The main types of social scripting include:

- quick-script
- SF story
- social album
- social interactive adventure

More minor variations of social scripting include:

- flyer
- cards
- ring-thing
- photo-fix

Different types of social scripts are used at different times and in different situations. In order to demonstrate the use of the various forms of social scripting let us set up a problem situation and go through it, step by step, employing a few of the forms listed above.

Problem Situation:

You are in a book store with your seven-year-old son, a youngster with a more mild form of autism. You have come to purchase a book for him which he had previously seen at that store. The book is no longer on the bookshelf in which it had last been seen, and the youngster is immediately alarmed.

"Somebody stole my book," says the youngster a bit too loudly.

"No, no, sweetheart. Perhaps the book was put someplace else," you respond, knowing full well that the book has probably been sold. Nevertheless, in the hope that somewhere within the walls of the store there rests another copy, you tell your youngster you will now ask the clerk to find the book.

Your youngster does not understand why the book is no longer there. The book had been there. It is no longer there. That sums it up for him!

"Somebody stole my book," he repeats, talking even louder. Like the earthquake, of sorts, the child is not able to cope with the disappointment of the missing book. It is more than he or she can bear. He places his bent arm over his head and begins to pace. Perhaps, in his or her mind there may never be another copy of it anywhere in the universe. It has been stolen and with its theft he is left in an unfair world over which he continues to have no control.

You run to the nearest clerk. He tells you that he has no more copies of that book. He tells you that he can bring a copy over from the warehouse. It will be there tomorrow. Or, he suggests you visit another branch of their store where there are copies of the book on the shelf.

You offer your child the opportunity to visit this other bookstore to find the missing book. Unfortunately the youngster is already consumed by the immediate overwhelming disappointment of a bookshelf with a space where this book should have been. Perhaps inside himself he is bewildered, puzzled, frightened. You had failed to control the entire world for him. Anxiety-ridden and angry it is apparent to you that he will soon lash out uncontrollably. A tantrum is underway.

Too late to recover you have a new goal; how to get the youngster out of the store and into the car as quickly as possible, before every eye in the store has refocused in your direction and on this child.

Through the eyes of this child perhaps we could see this incident a bit differently. This child may not understand why the book is missing. He probably does not understand the function and workings of a bookstore. He does not know how a bookstore operates. In his mind the book was his. It was just housed there. It was only waiting in this store for him to come and purchase it. It should have been there. It isn't. Therefore, something is terribly wrong. Its disappearance coupled with his inability to understand the way in which a bookstore works leave him, once again, in a world in which he has no control. In a confusing world, a world to which he may be overly sensitized, a world in which things move, appear and disappear without understanding, any loss can be more than he can bear.

We cannot control every facet of the world for this individual. And since we cannot control every facet of our environment, the problem of obtaining something he wants needs to be approached in another way. We need to find a way to enable the individual at risk, in this case the seven year old child with autism, to understand in advance, before we go into a store how a book store operates. He needs to understand that any item desired may or may not be available. Yet, if what he wants is not there, it can be ordered. He needs to understand that this is only one of many bookstores with many books. Just because one store does not have a book does not mean the book is not available. It just means that book is unavailable in that particular store on that particular day, at that particular moment. You can then present him with alternatives, should the book not be where he last saw it. You can take him to another store to find the book or you can order the book at this store. Then all he need do is write down on his calendar when the book will come to the store so that he can accompany you to claim it for his own. The important thing here is to prepare the child before you leave your home or your car.

Yet, you cannot always know what is in the mind of another individual. You may have no idea that at some previous time he had seen a given book, a book that he now wants. In this case a quiet bookstore can become the backdrop for a tantrum, unless you are able to do some pretty fast maneuvering. What kind of maneuvering?

If you, the parent, are cognizant of your child's initial reaction, you may be able to rescue the situation with the use of only a pencil and paper. By the use of Social Facilitation you can quickly outline the problem as your child sees it. Your written words and phrases can visually show your child that you share in his disappointment. However, you can let him know, succinctly, quickly, in outline form how the situation can be resolved to his satisfaction.

The written form can take several shapes. We call these social facilitative techniques "social scripting." Social scripting can come in many shapes. In this case, the quick script is the ideal solution. What method you use will depend upon the situation in which you find yourself. In the situation above, a timely and appropriate quick script might save the day. The script need not be long nor neat. It would, however, need to cover a few essential things.

It should:

- Be a concrete outline of the problem at hand.

- Provide a framework for obtaining the desired results.

- Validate the child's feelings of disappointment so as to reduce possible anxiety and/or anger.

Had you known about the desired book before entering the store you could have written out an SF story in advance of your visit. That story would have revealed possible alternatives, should the goal have been unattainable. As we previously mentioned, if the child, student or client understands the meaning behind a bookstore and the books within, if he understands that books appear, disappear and can reappear, if he understands that other stores may have this book and you have only to go and find it, a tantrum may be less likely to develop.

However, like most of us, you most probably didn't think this far ahead. Now what? Arming yourself with a quick script pad and pen or just an ordinary mid-size scratch pad and pen, you could write out the bare essentials of the situation and alternative solutions. A child used to seeing a quick script may look on quickly as you write, hoping to gain some insight, some understanding. If this is the case, the individual may be able to help make the decision involving what to do next.

If you can get the child's attention before the youngster is enmeshed in the tantrum, you may be able to deflect or prevent one by the use of the quick-script. The quick script is fast, fearless and hopefully fruitful. It is a stopgap measure to maintain decorum and control in a potentially explosive situation.

A quick script for this situation might be as simple as follows:

I am sad.
The Bubblegum book is gone.

The man wants to help me.
The man is happy.
He will get me a Bubblegum book in two days.
I will write two days on my calendar.
Then I can come to the bookstore and get my book.
Then I can take the Bubblegum book home.
I can put it in my room.
I am happy.
See you soon Bubblegum book.
The end!

Note the quick-script style used here. If the individual can refer to himself using the word "I", then you write in first person. If the individual refers to himself by name, you would phrase the story using third person. The individual is your key. Any work created must be in terms he understands and at his level. The social script created is short, concrete, to the point and complete. It does not condemn. It does not make a lot of judgement calls. It presents the problem, the facts, and a workable, concrete solution. It helps guide an emotional response.

Obviously, if the individual is already in an emotional tailspin telling him he's happy is not going to work. So, it behooves you, the social facilitator, to recognize and write out a solution as quickly as possible. Your goal is to get the individual to recognize the problem and buy into the solution, while recognizing and validating his position.

While there are other means to prevent or ward off a potential tantrum, the quick script provides an individual with a new understanding of that situation. Those other means specifically include the flyer and cards, the ring-thing and the photo-fix.

The flyer is just a one-page piece of paper that you may want to laminate (if it is to be used over a period of time). On the piece of paper you might have a schedule for a special activity or a new recipe for cookies. The flyer might be a map of a new school or a map of a library. Like Dumbo and his feather, the flyer can be a godsend.

Cards are a variation of a flyer. How many times have we seen cards that have a key word or math problem on one side and the definition or answer on the other? They can help the individual remember what comes first in a conversation, what comes second, third, etc. Cards can be a reminder. Cards can educate.

A "ring-thing" is usually made of three to four laminated flyers with a hole through a corner of one side. The sheets of the ring-thing are connected by a metal ring (somewhat like a large ring you might use for a key chain). The ring-thing can help an individual at home or away from home. Like the cards or the individual flyer, the various laminated pages usually contain pictures of things that are familiar, of interest and comforting to that individual. The ring-thing can be used anytime.

The "photo fix" could be a very small photo album you find in a stationery store. However, it should have room for a few words or phrases along with the pictures. It can be filled with pictures of some hobby that the individual enjoys. It should be a visual source of comfort. The photo fix is not necessarily a tool for education. It is a tool for redirection. It attempts to change the subject so that the individual is able to refocus his attention to something more soothing and comforting. When all else fails, or when you don't have time to write out a quick script, the photo fix can help.

However, if you were privy, in advance, to the knowledge that this youngster had a given goal at that store, you might have had time to create a short SF story to cover a possible problem situation. Below we have written out an example of an SF story for use in this kind of situation. Keep in mind that this is just one example. There are an infinite number of variations that can be created. You need only think about what is needed and write it out. We have provided a few possible examples.

SF Story Example One:

Mommy and I are going to the bookstore. I want to get the Bubblegum book at the bookstore. If the first bookstore has the Bubblegum book, Mommy will buy it for me. If the first bookstore does not have the Bubblegum book Mommy can order the Bubblegum book so that I can have it a different day. Or, Mommy and I can go to another bookstore to find the Bubblegum book. Mommy says I can decide if we will go to another store to find the Bubblegum book or ask the man to get me a Bubblegum book from this store.

The end

SF Story Example Two:

Mommy and I will go into the bookstore together. A bookstore is a quiet place. It is quiet like a library. I need to use my quiet voice in a bookstore. Mommy needs to use her quiet voice in the bookstore too.

We will look for the Bubblegum book. If the store does not have the Bubblegum book we can ask someone that works in the store to get me one. Or, Mommy and I can go to another bookstore to find the Bubblegum book. If I want to wait for a Bubblegum book to come to this store, I can come back and get it in a few days. I can write the new day to come on my calendar.

When the book gets to the store, the people will put my name on the book. This means the book is just for me. Then they will telephone our house and tell us to come and buy our Bubblegum book.

The people at the bookstore and my Mommy are helping me. They want me to have the Bubblegum book. When my Bubblegum book comes to the bookstore I will be very happy. See you soon Bubblegum book.

The end!

Having set up a sample of some type in this way and having read it at home with the youngster, the child is now armed with information. He knows you want to buy him the Bubblegum Book. He understands that though the book was last seen at the bookstore it may not be there today. In this way, if there is no Bubblegum Book on the shelf, he knows he will get one soon. It will be his book.

You could have written out a different script, a different SF story; one which indicated that we would visit a second store and even a third, if that is what you plan to do. You could have lengthened this one. You could have suggested something different to do, something fun. Some ideas for fun might mean go for ice cream, play video games, go to see a movie, rent a film, etc.

Perhaps your youngster has had difficulties previously when visiting a bookstore. Perhaps it was difficult to manage him or get him to leave when it was time to go home. Given the fact that your past experience with him might have been less than satisfactory, you may want to write a story like this one.

SF Story Example Three:

On Wednesday Mommy and I are going to go to the bookstore. I like to go to the bookstore. The bookstore is fun. There are many, many books in the bookstore. I like to look at the books. There are big books and little books. There are books with many pictures inside. There are books with no pictures inside. These books just have words.

The books in the bookstore belong to the store. The books in the bookstore do not belong to me. But I can look at the books in the bookstore. If I want to take one home I can ask Mommy to buy it for me. I can quietly say, "Mommy, will you please buy me this book?" If Mommy says no, maybe she will buy it for me on a different day. If Mommy says yes, we can buy the book. When we buy the book we give money to the man or lady who works at the store. The money pays for the book. Then we can take the book home. I can take the book into my room and sit down on my bed and read it. Going to the bookstore can make me feel good. Going to the bookstore is fun, especially when I am a good listener and a good whisperer.

The end

One of the many advantages of the SF story and its use prior to the potential experience is that if the individual is not happy with the SF story you will know in advance of your journey. You can then modify the words to meet an eventuality as well as his needs. The story can even be a joint venture, making him part of the creative SF story process, by asking for his input. Remember, the greater his understanding of a potential situation, the greater his interest in this process, the greater the chance for success.

The last form of social script addressed here is the social album. Usually written for a child whose reading skills are not as yet highly developed, the album is much like the SF story. However, the social album usually incorporates several photos and/or drawings. It also uses far fewer words and is generally much simpler and more straightforward in context and content. The photos usually reflect circumstances and situations with which the individual is familiar. Like you and I, most individuals enjoy seeing themselves in photographs. They especially enjoy seeing themselves in photographs in which they are successful or the situation is familiar and comforting. The saying, "one picture is worth a thousand words" applies especially well to this format. A social album, like a photograph album, usually has one or two photographs on a page with anywhere from one to five or six phrases or sentences. The words are direct and concrete. They come straight to the point. For the situation with the bookstore we might create an album as follows:

Bookstores have books.
I like books.

(leave sufficient space between paragraphs and place a snapshot of books in a store here)

I like words.
I like pictures.
Bookstores are quiet inside.

(leave sufficient space between paragraphs and place a photo of the inside of a bookstore here)

My classroom at school is quiet.

(leave sufficient space between paragraphs and place a photo of the inside of a classroom here)

I can use my whisper voice in school.

(leave sufficient space between paragraphs and place a photo of a child with happy face here)

I need to use my whisper voice in the bookstore.

Quiet voices in a bookstore make people happy.
If I use my quiet voice I can whisper words.
Can I have the book, Mommy?
I can show Mommy my book.
Maybe Mommy will buy it for me.
Thank you Mommy.
Thank you bookstore.
I am happy.

(leave sufficient space and place a picture of a Happy Face here)

(leave sufficient space and place a photo of child holding a book here)

The job of a Social Facilitator is simply to facilitate better social understanding. The facilitator seeks to accomplish this understanding through the creation of various kinds of social scripting, like the ones we developed. These social scripts include carefully written social clues and cues. Concepts are broken down into logical basic components. These components help to enable individuals to grasp meanings previously missing. Peer behavior, the meaning behind an action, the use of specific props all can become better understood. Even the social album, seemingly simple in context and concept can have great meaning to a youngster or other individual at risk.

The Social Facilitation process relies on careful observation of the child or other individual at risk within the specific social settings where that person has difficulties. The process involves consultations with key players. If you are a parent, teacher, therapist, doctor, nurse, classroom aide or peer of those that need help, you are one of these key players. You can provide valuable insight into the strengths and weaknesses exhibited by the individual at risk in a given situation.

The social facilitative technique used should be designed to help the individual at risk broaden his or her panorama. The quick script, SF story or social album to be created should be designed to provide a clear, finite, definitive, comfort-inducing, anxiety-reducing framework to help the individual modify his or her behavior. It will need to be positive, logical and encouraging. It should seek to reduce negative and maladaptive words and behaviors by concretely providing positive, alternative, concrete solutions.

Remember our actor Joe on Neptune, the one we left alone with the green goo givers? Now Joe, social script in hand, being greeted by those strange Neptunians, having prior knowledge that goo-giving is the Neptunian way of saying "Aloha," can develop a suitable and appropriate response. Indeed, if he possessed the information within a written script, he most probably would have brought some green goo of his own to distribute, thus behaving in an acceptable, appropriate way.

Whether the individual at risk is mildly, moderately or severely impaired, it is our belief that social scripting is an important tool, a tool that can make a difference in the lives of those we seek to help.

The most important thing to remember is that we are all unique, cut from innumerable molds, seeing a finite world through infinite perspectives. It behooves us to help each other so that we create a common ground for understanding, a common worldliness for and with each other. A part of the job of you, the social facilitator, is to help that individual in need understand that other people may not see the world precisely the way he or she does and that our job is to help him see the world in a similar way. Be the differences Autism or Asperger's Syndrome, Obsessive-Compulsive Disorder or Tourette Syndrome, Bi-Polar Disorder or ADD, or any other catchall category, we believe Social Facilitation can and will make a difference.

Chapter X

A World of Difference

I say something to you. You respond, saying something back to me. In this exchange of words perhaps we are trying to give each other something. A question arises. Is what I am attempting to communicate to you the same thing as what you interpret from me? Is there complete shared meaning behind our exchange of words? The answer to this question is most probably no. You and I would derive different interpretations, differing meaning, behind the words we share. Certainly our body language might help enable us to more fully understand one another, yet each of us would ultimately comprehend a situation a bit differently. How could it be otherwise? We are two completely different people with different past histories and different past experiences. Each of us is truly unique, genetically unique, and culturally unique. No two of us could have possibly experienced life identically. The experiences I have had, in the order in which I have had them and under the circumstances in which I have had them are going to have been different from yours.

Add to this mix genetics, culture and experience and we quickly come to realize that any possibility of a totally shared linguistic, emotional and intellectual understanding is ludicrous. Even if we were clones of one another, genetically identical, our placement in the womb would begin to experientially separate us long before birth, thus affecting our future perception and attitude toward every future event.

The more different we are from one another culturally, experientially and genetically, the more likely we would be to perceive and derive a different meaning from the words of each other. Even a dictionary definition will be interpreted differently by each of us because we come to the dictionary with our own uniqueness.

Let me give you an example. A small meteor suddenly crashes through the roof of my car parked below on the street. As the car smolders I sit, unaware of the incident, inside my office having a salami sandwich. The meteor destroys my car. What is my understanding of this experience? How might I explain the mishap to others? What impact might this event have on my understanding of life and the workings of the universe? Could I explain this event in such a way as to enable another to understand the event precisely as I do? Here again, the answer is probably no. I cannot provide you, through word or gesture, a precise understanding of the experience I just had. Even if you tried to put yourself in my place your own background would cause you to see, feel, understand, and ultimately respond to the event in your own unique way.

It isn't just the words, my friends, that we each understand uniquely, but the concepts as well. Any shared understanding of some concept is, at best, similar.

Indeed, we come from all over the globe. We have different siblings, relatives, friends and teachers. We have lived in different environments, different places, at various points in history. Our lives have been different. Our experiences have been different. If we add to these factors the problems associated with developmental difficulties and disabilities, we compound the difficulty of transcending differences.

Let me tell you about something that happened recently. Our older son came to us worried about someone he has known since childhood. "He has no self-confidence," said my twenty-three year-old son referring to this twenty-eight year-old friend with whom he works. "He won't try anything new. I think he is afraid he'll fail. He's so smart. I know he can do the work, but he won't even try. He just becomes volatile, even hostile. Sometimes he even thinks people are talking about him behind his back. Of course we're not. I just don't understand. I just can't seem to get through to him. He just kind of shuts himself off from me, from everyone."

Having known the young man to whom my son was referring since childhood these words did not surprise me. It is unfortunate that no one has ever recognized his difficulties. It is a shame that he has spent a lifetime trying desperately to find a way to cope with serious challenges. He has managed to grow up and face a world in which he is somewhat unprepared and has spent a good deal of his life feeling frustrated and overwhelmed. And, when no longer able to hold his emotions in check, he has lashed out.

I have seen this young man in action. He is a whiz with a computer, a genius of sorts. His knowledge of computers, their design and application, his navigation and understanding of the Internet is mind-boggling. Given the time to explore and learn on his own, at his own pace, his genius becomes apparent. Given the time to explore in his own way, he becomes another person, happy, bubbly, and contented.

How can he be helped? How do we respond to a human being, adult or child, with special needs so that his needs can be met comfortably and appropriately, making use of strengths, not weaknesses? How can we disarm potentially explosive situations in a beneficial way, a way that best promotes understanding while keeping fears, anxieties, confusion and the need to shut down or withdraw in check? Take a look at the following imaginary oral exchange between an adult (Mother) and her son (Johnny), whom we shall identify as having been previously diagnosed with either Asperger's Syndrome or high-functioning autism.

Child: "What happened to Buggie? Did he fall into the abyss?"

Adult: "Who is Buggie?"

Child: "What happened to him?"

Adult: "I don't know who Buggie is. Is he a cartoon character?"

Child: "Did Buggie fall into the abyss? Huh? Huh?"

Adult: "Who is Buggie?"

Child: "He's on television. What happened to him?"

Adult: "I'm sorry, sweetie. I've never seen or heard of Buggie. Is he a cartoon character?"

Child: "Is he in the abyss? Huh? Huh?"

Adult: "It's okay sweetheart. I'm sure ..."

Child: "Oh no! My poor Buggie is hurt. He's dead!"

Adult: "It's okay sweetheart. I'm sure Buggie will be fine."

Child: "Tell me! Tell me!"

Obviously the character "Buggie" is not real, but this kind of response by this type of child most probably is. Perhaps a verbal exchange, such as this one, is not totally unfamiliar to you. And, in fact, a situation like this one might easily progress or escalate into a confrontation or tantrum. If so, why? Why is this scenario so unacceptable, so threatening to this child?

I believe it is problematic because the adult and child are not connecting. The responses of the adult are not meeting the needs of the child. The expectation of help from the adult is not materializing. Therefore the fears and anxieties held by the child remain unresolved. What is also apparent is that the child holds the adult responsible to have all answers to all questions at all times. And thirdly, what is also apparent is that the adult is unable to communicate to this child the fact that she has no prior knowledge of this television program.

The adult communicated to the child in the way most of us do, orally. The entire exchange was oral and it was ineffectual. The adult spoke words to a child filled with emotion, a child who might have needed more than mere words could provide him. Finding these words, presented in the way in which they were, of little help or comfort, his apprehensions began to multiply. His mother probably felt a sense of inadequacy coupled with a foreboding of what might come next. How can this change?

Getting back to our imaginary scenario, young Johnny now has one arm draped over his head, bent at the elbow, while his other arm is butted up against his cheek. Beginning to pace, like a caged tiger, all the while drawing closer to his mother, his mother becomes more aware of Johnny's heightened level of anxiety.

Until now we have said that the "explanation," the "defense," the "response" of the adult has been oral. Yet, we can easily see that if something does not change, this interaction could further deteriorate. However, we might halt the emotional slide if we change the *mode of its delivery*. The mode of delivery which we believe will best resolve this problem, the mode of delivery which might easily bring it to a fruitful conclusion would initially be a "quick-script." The quick-script could be considered a first line of defense, a Band-Aid, of sorts. It is a stopgap measure, written on the spot as need arises. It is an important form of Social Facilitation. It can be an effective treatment to keep a potentially stormy encounter from turning into a full-fledged hurricane, enabling calm seas to prevail. It has the potential to neutralize and stabilize a situation. With its use, the needs of this child might be better addressed. With its use, information not readily able to be auditorily assimilated in a timely manner might be assimilated faster and with better understanding.

Let us, therefore, expand upon this hypothetical interaction, using the "quick-script."

Adult: "Let's write about Buggie together. Would Johnny like that?"

Child: "Yes."

Adult: (Taking note that the child is following close in tow his mother moves slowly and calmly, picking up a pencil and pad)

We'll continue the quick-script a bit further on. Right now we need to note the emotional level of Johnny's mother. She has a special responsibility here. She must remain totally calm. In fact, the more upset Johnny appears to become, the calmer she will need to be. If she allows herself to become agitated, her emotional level may only exacerbate the situation. It is our belief that many of these individuals at risk respond to the emotional level of others. Indeed, they appear to almost take on the physical manifestation of the emotional level of those around them, in this case Johnny's mother. Perhaps this is one of the reasons why it can be difficult to take these individuals into crowded situations. They become emotionally over-stimulated, unable to handle all the stimuli surrounding them, perhaps even taking on the emotional "vibes" they pick up. This might not be as far-fetched as one might think. After all, if we accept the premise that many of these individuals appear to be overly sensitive to sound, touch, smell and sight, what prevents them from being overly sensitive to some kind of emotional stimulation radiating out from others? And, if this is so, how awful it must be for them; unable to understand what they perceive, ignore it or ward it off. Johnny's mother must keep her cool. The more upset Johnny appears to be, the calmer she needs to remain.

Rule #1: A pencil and pad should always be handy. In fact, you may want to keep a few pencils and pads scattered about the house so that if a problem arises, you are always ready to write. Our adult in this scenario begins to write. She writes as succinctly, briefly and as quickly as possible, because this child, like so many other individuals at risk, needs, craves, demands resolution and closure to his dilemma. And he needs it NOW!

The mother in our scenario knows that this problem cannot remain unresolved. To do so would be tantamount to abandoning the emotional needs of her son. Johnny must make sense of the senseless, derive meaning and gain understanding so that he can move on.

If we were to look at the situation at hand a bit closer, we could note that on one side is the child in need while on the other side is an unresolved and confusing situation, one which he might think not only unpleasant but unfair as well. The adult, in this case Johnny's mother, is in the middle. She is perceived as an all-knowing conduit, the link, the fulcrum who must, somehow, both balance and connect the two sides; and thus bring harmony through understanding. In this scenario it is the task of Johnny's mother to close the gap, providing a connecting bridge of understanding. And that first connection, the first Band-Aid is our quick-script.

Our main character in the scenario, Johnny, might choose to follow along, because he cannot wait. He will watch you develop the script, perhaps even read over your shoulder as you write. The material his mother develops, presented visually, logically, and sequentially may be all that is needed. This concrete solution then becomes a bridge between child, adult, and problem. Not only does this bridge represent a connection, but also, just as importantly and perhaps even more importantly, the child becomes aware that the adult understands his problem. He is not alone, stranded, left to flounder and worry. He has been able to garner the support of the adult. They are socially interacting as well as solving a problem together.

The quick-script that his mother writes will concretely break down his dilemma into visual units that are on his level and which meet his needs. She writes the quick-script in real time. The level of understanding determines whether the quick-script will be written in third person using the individual's name, or in first person using the pronoun "I". For example, the mother could choose to write "Johnny is worried about Buggie," if he commonly refers to himself as Johnny, or "I am worried about Buggie," if he commonly refers to himself using the pronoun "I". In this case we'll call Johnny by name.

In our imaginary scenario, the quick-script involves Johnny's mother, Johnny and Buggie, the cartoon character. The way the scenario has been set up there is no way Mommy could know anything that transpired in the cartoon. Maybe she was baking a cherry cheesecake. Maybe she was taking a nap. For whatever reason, she was not privy to the cartoon. She begins to create the quick-script.

Adult: "Johnny is worried about Buggie. Mommy knows that Johnny wants Buggie to be okay. Mommy wants Buggie to be okay too. Can we say that Buggie will get out of the abyss? Can we write Buggie a letter telling him that he can climb out of the abyss and be okay?"

Child: "Can Buggie be better? Can we write to him now?"

Adult: "Yes, Johnny. Let's write him a letter now. Would you like to write the letter or would you like Mommy to write the letter?"

Child: "You write it."

Adult: (Mommy takes a sheet of paper and begins to write)

Dear Buggie,
Johnny wants you to be better. He wants you to get out of the abyss. An abyss is a deep, dark hole. You can climb out. Then you will be okay. Then you will be safe.

(Mommy seals the letter in an envelope, addresses it to the television station and places a stamp on it. Together, she and Johnny go to the nearest mailbox and Johnny puts the letter inside. Situation resolved!)

Let's stop here for a moment. Johnny has probably become calmer. This is because he is beginning to perceive that he has some control in the situation. The environment is not manipulating him through Buggie. Instead, he is in control. He has found a way to save Buggie. The world is no longer unfair. All is becoming right with the world. Buggie will be safe, thanks to Johnny. He has concretely provided Buggie with a way to escape disaster. Johnny has taken a proactive role. The letter has saved the situation!

We can stop here. We have disarmed the explosive moment. Note that his mother could have created a longer quick-script, one that could have been more in depth. However, Johnny's momentary needs were met successfully. To have gone on and on might not have accomplished anything further and could have put him on overload. Taking this fact into consideration his mother might have decided to delve a bit further into her son's lack of understanding. She might later decide to create something a bit more encompassing, something a bit deeper, something that will give Johnny a better understanding of the world around him. His mother might take a bit of time and develop an SF story. We use the SF story as a second form of Social Facilitation.

SF Story:

Yesterday Johnny was sad. He was watching Buggie on television. Buggie was in the abyss and Johnny was worried. Johnny thought Buggie was gone forever. Johnny thought Mommy saw the Buggie movie. But Mommy did not see the movie like Johnny did. Mommy was busy when Johnny was watching the Buggie movie. Mommy was in the kitchen. Mommy was baking a cherry cheesecake while Johnny was watching the Buggie movie. Mommy was in the kitchen; Johnny was in the family room. The television is in the family room. There is no television to see Buggie in the kitchen. Mommy could not hear the Buggie movie. Mommy could not see the Buggie movie. Only Johnny could see the Buggie movie. Only Johnny could hear the Buggie movie.

Can Johnny see the television when he is in the kitchen? No. Johnny cannot see the television when he is in the kitchen. Can Johnny hear the television when he is in the kitchen? No. Johnny cannot hear the television when he is in the kitchen. When Mommy is in the kitchen and Johnny is in the family room watching television Johnny can see and hear the television. The kitchen is far away from the family room. The walls stop Mommy from seeing the television when she is in the kitchen. The sounds of the television are far away from Mommy when she is in the kitchen and Johnny is watching television in the family room. So Mommy cannot see or hear the television when she is cooking or baking in the kitchen.

When Johnny watches Buggie on television Johnny should come and ask Mommy to come and watch the television with him. Then Mommy and Johnny can talk about Buggie. Then Mommy and Johnny can share words and ideas. Then Mommy and Johnny can talk about Buggie together. Then we can help each other. Johnny can ask Mommy questions and Mommy can answer. Then Mommy asks Johnny questions and he can answer. When Mommy and Johnny watch television together and share words and ideas together they have fun. Sharing questions and answers is fun. Learning is fun. Sharing can make us happy. Let's be happy.

Note that the original quick-script was quite short. It was just long enough to defuse a potentially unpleasant confrontation. It introduced a united attempt to solve a problem. Following this encounter, Johnny's mother decided to take the situation a bit further by trying to get Johnny to understand why she had initially been unable to help him. She went on to explain to him what happens when we do different things at the same time. She took it even a step further by providing an opportunity to teach Johnny a little bit about sharing. The initial situation provided the opportunity to create an SF story to learn a bit about what makes us happy. Even if Johnny does not thoroughly comprehend or seems unable to grasp all that his mother has presented, we never know how much will be absorbed now, how much will be useful later and what impact the entire sequence has had on him. It remains to be seen. The quick-script can be a jumping off point from which a good SF story can later develop.

That story has certain essential characteristics. It must be logical and sequential and meaningful. The SF story is to be written as if you were doing a geometry proof taking the reader, step by step, through a confusing maze and into the light of understanding. The piece you create draws to a logical conclusion.

Taking a closer look at both the quick-script and the SF story, note that they both make use of many descriptive statements. Note too that these sentences address feelings in a carefully worded way, matching feeling with task without overloading the reader. We use what we believe to be the child's emotional state. Harkening back to Goleman's work, we are reminded that these children are often unable to put a label on how they feel.

We believe that if we can provide them with a written word or name to identify how they feel, we may help them identify and put a name to an emotion or group of emotions held within. In the future, perhaps the individual at risk may begin to be able to call forth this word to identify how he feels. If, however, we write out a word that does not match some internal definition for that word, perhaps we may be lucky enough to get corrected. Better to risk being wrong and continue the dialogue than to not even attempt to help.

What we need to remember is that we are trying to understand the world through their eyes so that we can help expand upon that world, bringing it more akin to our own understanding. We are providing a rack to hang a hat on! If our rack is not the right one, perhaps they will help us create the right one.

We expanded upon the quick-script by the development and use of the SF story. We used the story to demonstrate why Mommy was unable to initially help Johnny. That explanation was an attempt to separate Johnny from his Mother. "You did X while I did Y. You did not know what I was doing and I was not party to what you were doing. You were here and I was there. If you need me to hear and see what you hear and see then I must be with you." This concretely helps to show Johnny why his mother did not initially understand his problem. This helps Johnny separate from his mother. This may help him begin to understand that they are distinct and separate entities with separate and distinct perspectives.

Yet Johnny's mother let him know that she cared about his dilemma and wanted to help resolve it. By doing this she added a connecting touch of empathy to the pot, something children like Johnny often appear to lack, but in reality, may not lack in abundance or at all. Through our words and deeds we seek to model or demonstrate empathy for them. Their dilemma or problem is then broken down to its basic components and succinctly written out. We answer all possible "why" questions and provide the "how to" directives.

In other words, we give them written ingredients, what these ingredients look like and what they do. This method, this recipe, is in no way random. It is a way to engage mother and son in a conversation about Buggie once again, some time in the future. The story could have gone on and on. It could have talked about other television characters and other television programs. What may appear as a rather boring hodgepodge group of sentences is, in essence, a "how to" recipe, a recipe written "in concrete," on paper.

Another way to put it is to compare this material to a kind of geometry problem. This approach can give this individual a formula to once again engage his mother, or some significant other, in some past dilemma. It gives him a way to engage in a conversation about something he might continue to find interesting. Indeed, the next time Buggie or another cartoon or program attracts his interest and he wants his mother to be part of the experience, he might recognize the fact that he has a concrete way to achieve his goal. He need only ask his mother to go into the television room and watch the program with him. Perhaps his ability to generalize may not come as quickly as we would like, but over time, and with repeated quick-script and SF story intervention, the technique can provide him with a viable way to meet his needs and achieve his goals.

Something else took place within the scope of this quick-script and SF story sequence. Johnny's mother let him know that she wanted to be included in his interests whenever he would allow her. In addition, she gave him a recipe to make it happen. In no way was this quick-script/SF story combination random. It was calculated, organized, logical and sequential. Let's go through it once again from another perspective.

"Johnny is sad." We gave Johnny a word that is familiar yet will probably not propel him into further action. In contrast, a word like "angry" might. Yet we have done more. We gave a name to Johnny's amorphous state, we have given him permission to own it and know it and we have aligned his emotion with a word that defines it. Since Johnny did not balk at his Mother's use of the word "sad," she continues to write. If sad was not an acceptable word Johnny might have been able to yell out a substitute word like "upset." If, however, "sad" is adequate or "upset" is labeled as better by Johnny, then perhaps the match between emotion and word may have given him a means of calming himself as his mother continues to work toward resolution to his problem.

Since, however, Johnny did not volunteer a substitute word, we might assume that either the word sad met his needs or that he was unable to come up with another choice or that the word made no impact on him. He continued to read.

If Johnny was a bit more ready and in control, we could have given him a broader choice of terms, even gambling on more potentially emotionally loaded ones such as disappointed, frustrated, or mad.

His Mother even gave him a second emotion. She said she thought he was worried about Buggie and that she knows Johnny wants Buggie to be okay. Certainly Johnny did not say these things to his Mother. She is attempting to match action and emotion with words. She both acknowledges and defines what she witnesses. She aligns emotion with word. She defines where before there were only amorphous feelings of uneasiness.

Mommy has done something else. She has let Johnny know that she also has feelings, that these feelings may be the same or different from his, that she recognizes and acknowledges his feelings and that she cares about them. Oftentimes I am convinced that many, if not most of these individuals, are not fully aware that we are separate and distinct entities. This makes it important to draw boundaries between us and those we seek to help. Johnny's mother demonstrates this as she goes on to acknowledge that she too felt badly about Buggie's dilemma; she as a separate entity. Further, Mommy let Johnny know that together, as a team, they could solve the dilemma.

The SF story gave Johnny a reason why his mother could not completely understand his frustrations with Buggie's situation. Mommy was baking in one room while Johnny was watching television in another. Next, we concretely describe the reason why his mother could not accommodate his request by telling him that baking in the kitchen prevents her from seeing and hearing the television. In fact, it might be useful for Mommy to demonstrate physically why she cannot hear or see the television from the kitchen. If Johnny were willing, she could physically take Johnny into the kitchen and demonstrate the problem. It is crucial that at some point Johnny begin to understand that his mother cannot be privy to everything that he sees, hears or experiences unless she is with him. At some point it will be necessary for him to begin to understand that his mother is a distinct, separate entity.

Yet, his mother did something more. She let Johnny know that she was doing something for him, when she was away from him. She was doing something from which he will later derive pleasure. She was baking a cherry cheesecake. In this way Johnny might begin to understand that Mommy was not ignoring his needs, but was meeting different needs, other needs. It also gives her a way to segue into another arena. That of food!

Lastly, his mother gives him a way to get his future needs met. The next time this cartoon or a different one presents itself on television he can come and ask his mother to join him and watch the program. He is told that together he and his mother can watch a show that he finds interesting. His mother has given him a recipe for sharing his interest.

The end of the scene is pleasant and positive. It provides warm words and ideas. And how did we do it all? We did it by:

- Reducing complicated material to discrete units of understanding.
- Using words and pictures to break down barriers of confusion.
- Using words and pictures to rebuild with understanding.

Whether Johnny was looking for answers, comfort, interaction, or all three, we still do not know. What we do know is that we used all three to try and resolve a fearful and anxiety-producing situation.

If we can develop and use quick-scripts, SF stories, and albums and build from them, recognizing new areas of need, then more growth might be in the making. And that is our goal.

Chapter XI

The Quick Script Model "QS"
(The Crisis Mode)

In Chapter IX we talked about many things, including a focus on the different modes of Social Facilitation. Within this chapter we will look more closely at the quick script, its development and use, along with some examples. We will also introduce the quick script pad and its neighbor, the quick script schedule pad.

A quick script can be written, using pad and pen, wherever you are and whenever the need arises. A problem can suddenly develop just as you were about to leave the home; or one can quite suddenly rear its head when you are out and about, anywhere, everywhere. The quick script is a stopgap measure. It can be damage control at its best! It is:

- simple
- quick
- logical
- meaningful
- told through the eyes of the individual at risk

It is used to prevent a volatile situation from erupting. It is used to help the individual at risk understand a potentially difficult or upsetting situation. It is used is to quell any disappointment or anxiety brought about by some unforeseen problem.

As we have said previously, you need only a pen and quick script pad, or any writing implement and writing pad, to help the differently abled individual. It is the words, phrases and sentences you use that will make a difference. You can write on an envelope or even a paper napkin, if necessary.

Sometimes we can make use of other written forms, forms we have already talked about, such as the flyer or cards, the photo-fix or ring-thing. We use whatever works.

Below you will find samples of a quick script and two flyers. Prior to each example we have described the situation that prompted the script or flyer's development.

The Quick Script

A five-year-old child with autism wakes up with a temperature, a cough, sniffles and red cheeks. Conclusion: He is sick. Remedy: He will need to go to doctor. Problem: In the past, going to the doctor has not been a pleasant experience. Not for the doctor, not for his office staff, not for the individual at risk and certainly not for his parents.

The doctor's office was called and an appointment made. Then, taking pencil and pad the following quick script would be written quickly. It would be written through the eyes of the child. It would be concrete and succinct using vocabulary with which he was familiar. It would be logical and sequential and would be linguistically similar in pattern to the way he spoke about himself. Because this child always referred to himself (at this age) using his name, the quick script would be written this way. The script would not admonish him. It would not tell him what to do. It would merely list pieces of data he needed in order to successfully complete a course of action. By telling him what would happen at the doctor's office we gave him time to prepare himself. There would be no surprises. He would be ready.

Quick Script Example:

Seth is coughing.
Seth is sneezing.
Seth is hot.
Seth has a temperature.
Seth is sick.
Seth needs to see the doctor.

The doctor helps children.
The doctor can help Seth.
The doctor will listen to Seth's heart.

The doctor will look in Seth's ears.
The doctor will look inside Seth's mouth.
The doctor will feel Seth's belly.
The doctor will give Seth medicine.

Then Seth will feel better.
Seth can have a lollypop.
Seth and Mommy will go home.

Following the development of the script I had the child sit next to me. I slowly and quietly read the words to him, pointing at each word as we went along. His eyes followed my finger. We then went through it a second time. I then gave him the story to hold as we got into the car and drove to the doctor's office.

He went quietly into the building. He went quietly into the doctor's office. He walked into the examining room, holding my hand. I lifted him onto the examining table. He sat quietly. The doctor came in and examined him following the course of action described on the quick script. He continued to sit quietly. Soon the doctor gave us a prescription, Seth got his lollypop and we were on our way. How different was his behavior from other children his age? On appearance, very little.

What had been done? We had given this child a tool. We had given him the opportunity to understand and prepare himself for the event to follow. The tool, the quick script, was a concrete, logical sequence of what was going to happen and why. Nothing negative was included in the script. When we entered the office this child knew what would happen. He had a concrete outline and time to emotionally prepare. He was privy to information, to a process that was to occur. The quick script does not need to contain everything. Just the basic facts. And it worked!

The Flyer

Shortly after the doctor visit, a call came in from the local elementary school. The special education teacher was having a problem with a six-year-old student. It seemed that he wanted the door and windows of the room closed at all times. Unfortunately, there was no air conditioning in the classroom and the days were becoming quite warm.

The teacher was concerned because more and more of her time was being consumed by opening the door after the child got up to close it. She would have to open the windows after he repeatedly got up to close them. The resulting situation often decayed into a meltdown by the student.

The remedy was not difficult, I told the teacher. Do the following. Take two sheets of paper. On one sheet write:

DOOR STAYS OPEN

[On the other sheet write:]

WINDOW STAYS OPEN

[Tape the one for the door on the door. Tape the one for the window on the window. That's all you need!]

Within an hour there was a second call from the teacher. She told me she was amazed. She said that after she taped the flyers as directed, the youngster went to the door, preparing to close it. But the sign said "Door stays open" so he returned to his chair. And each time he went to close the window the other sign said "Window stays open." Once again he returned to his seat.

Ladies and gentlemen, you don't have to be an Einstein to put Social Facilitation into action. The quick script and the flyers are just logical and straightforward. They merely require knowledge of the individual at risk. And if you are the parent, or caretaker, or teacher of this individual, you already know him well.

The few words in these flyers were all that was necessary to keep a potentially explosive situation from occurring. The concrete written word was law.

When you think about it, how different are we? If we read something in an article or book we believe it to be the truth, the whole truth and nothing but the truth. Is that not so? Why should the child at risk be any different? Is he any less gullible than we are?

By putting something visually in print we had helped him find meaning where there had previously been none.

When we hear a discussion on radio or watch people talking about an issue on television or network news, how much do we believe? Aren't we more likely to weigh this kind of information? Aren't we somewhat more likely to reject that which we might find questionable if it is not in print? I believe that just as our children might fail to absorb verbal information, the concretized written form can make the difference. In addition, in the written form we may have found a way to reveal a clearer picture of some of the profoundly complex intricate subtleties which social situations present.

Quick Script Pad

In chapter V we discussed a potentially problematic situation involving a youngster and his mother in an ice cream parlor. The flavor ice cream this youngster wanted was unavailable. Obviously, the mother had no way of knowing that this particular flavor would be unavailable. To demonstrate the potential use of a quick script pad in this situation, we have first provided you with a blank quick script pad form and then one filled in with the words the mother might use to ameliorate the situation.

Quick Script Pad

Identify Emotion(s): sad frustrated confused mad
disappointed angry bored hurt other __________________

Situation: Insert name/pronoun + emotion(s) + problem:

_________________________ feel(s) _______________________

because: ____

____

Getting Help (information):______________________________

____

____

____

List Options/Choices: ___________________________________

Action Taken: ____

Concluding Feelings: ______________________________________

Quick Script Pad

Identify Emotion(s): sad frustrated confused mad

disappointed angry bored hurt other ______________

Situation: Insert name/pronoun + emotion(s) + problem:

I feel(s) ***sad***

because: ***my chocolate chip ice cream is gone.***

Getting Help (information): ***The man says the chocolate chip ice cream will be here tomorrow at 1:00 p.m.***

List Options/Choices: ***I can get chocolate chip ice cream tomorrow. Today I can get a different flavor ice cream.***

Action Taken: ***I am going to get chocolate chunk ice cream today and chocolate chip ice cream tomorrow. I can write chocolate chip words on my calendar.***

Concluding Feelings: ***I am happy because I will have chocolate chip ice cream tomorrow.***

What about running errands? We all run them. And oftentimes our children go with us. Sometimes our missions run smoothly; at other times not so smoothly. That is why we developed the Quick Script Schedule Pad. Fill it out before you leave the house, leaving the "open" lines free of words. Follow the schedule, in order of items listed. If you suddenly need to make an unscheduled stop, write it down in the "open line" where it belongs so that the schedule remains orderly. The schedule gives the child or adult at risk information and time to prepare himself. Unscheduled and unwritten stops can be confusing and frustrating. The schedule pad can help. The application of the quick script schedule pad can lead to the successful completion of subsequent events or actions. Here is a blank quick script schedule pad:

Quick Script Schedule Pad

Day: ______________________________

Date: ______________________________

First Stop: ______________________________

Open: ______________________________

Next Stop: ______________________________

Open: ______________________________

Next Stop: ______________________________

Open: ______________________________

Next Stop: ______________________________

Open: ______________________________

Next Stop: ______________________________

A filled-in quick script schedule pad as a sample for you to see is show here:

Quick Script Schedule Pad

Day: ***Friday***

Date: ***March 10, 2000***

First Stop: ***Breakfast at Restaurant***

Open:____________________

Next Stop: ***Supermarket***

Open:____________________

Next Stop: ***Home***

Open:____________________

Next Stop: ***Dry Cleaner***

Open:____________________

Next Stop: ***Haircut***

Once again, you will notice that between each scheduled stop is an "Open" option. This is provided to provide flexibility in the schedule should a last minute need arise. For example, an unplanned stop at the gas station can be inserted as needed, with the updated schedule then shared with the individual in need. The pad can even be interactive. The parent can offer the special needs child the chance to add a local destination of their choice, and the parent and child can make a cooperative decision as to where to place their stops.

Whether you choose to use the quick script pad and its sister, the quick script schedule pad, is purely a personal decision. The two forms have been carefully created and made available to you to simplify your job. Whichever way you choose to go, with or without the pads, we believe the quick script concept is an essential tool in Social Facilitation.

Chapter XII

The Social Facilitation Story Model (SF Story)

"Your son hasn't learned one thing in physical education this year," he told me at the yearly, individualized educational programming meeting (IEP). "I have worked with him in groups and individually. He does not play baseball!"

I was shocked. The special education teacher went on to tell me that my then ten-year-old son was the worst player in either of the two classes he was working with. Furthermore, he wasn't sure my son even knew what the game was about.

"It's June. School ends in three weeks. Why wasn't I informed before the close of the year about this problem?" I asked. Nobody had an answer.

"He may not be playing baseball now," I said defensively, breaking the silence. "But, come next fall when school resumes I can assure you he will!"

I made an appointment to visit our son's fourth grade class. Early that morning I appeared, camera over the shoulder, pad and pencil in hand. I took several photos of my child and his behavior at the playing field. It was obvious that this child did not want to play. Why, I was not sure. I asked several questions of his classroom teacher and the class aides. I questioned my son, trying to figure out just why he was not taking part in the game. Within a short time I had the answer. He was not playing because he didn't have a clue what was going on and what his role was. All he knew was that this was his least favorite part of the day.

Over the next few days I developed the photo shots and created an SF story to meet what I felt were his current needs. The story would be a flash point, a starting point from which to move on to other areas.

Once the story was created with the photos of him in action with his classmates, we sat down together and read through the story. Because baseball is far more complicated than I had originally considered, the story was read over the course of the day. We read one chapter, then a second, then a third and lastly the fourth. The next day we went through it a second time.

What was particularly significant was the response of the child to the story. The story not only contained all the information one needed to know about baseball at school, but the photographs of him at the game along with the emotional feelings I gave him at the game seemed to make a difference.

Shortly thereafter he asked to go to a baseball game at the local stadium. His father talked and talked and talked to him during the game. He described what was happening. We had no idea what he was taking in and what was passing over his head.

A few days later our son asked if we would get him a baseball game for his Sega Genesis or his brother's Play Station. We immediately bought it. His older brother sat with him, hour after hour, helping him learn to bat and to field on the television screen. The ball was hit, the crowd cheered, the outfielder went after the ball and he ran toward first base. He became better and better.

Soon he was asking for a program to learn about professional baseball on the computer. Within a few weeks he knew the names of every player on the local team as well as the city, state and stadium names in which every baseball team, both American League and National League, played. He graced us with his enthusiasm and knowledge. No doubt about it, he was definitely becoming interested in baseball. And, more importantly, he was enjoying himself and feeling more confident. He happily asked if we could go to another game at the local stadium.

By the beginning of August he had requested a baseball cap, a ball, a bat and a glove from the local sports shop. Nothing could have made us happier. His father and brother shopped with him, getting him just the right equipment, as well as a little something for themselves. For the next several weeks we all got out there with him to play baseball. It was a family endeavor and it worked!

Come September we got a telephone call from the physical education teacher at school. He was shocked! "Not only is your son now playing baseball, he is the best, most enthusiastic player on his team," he said happily. "My only difficulty with him is that he only wants to play baseball. He won't play basketball. Can you help?"

"Yes, of course," I responded.

SF Story Example 1:

BASEBALL GAMES AT SCHOOL

Chapter 1

Sometimes our class plays baseball. When it is time to play baseball our teacher tells us to line up. I line up with my class. We go outside. We all walk together to the baseball diamond. I walk slowly because I don't want to play. I don't like to play baseball because I don't understand how to play baseball.

"Hurry up, Seth" my teachers call out to me. They don't understand that I don't want to play. But I do. I don't understand the rules in a baseball game. I don't know what I am supposed to do. Because I don't know how to play and don't understand the rules, I don't play baseball very well. That makes me feel bad.

When our class plays baseball I move away from everyone. I turn away. When I turn away I can't see the game or the kids. When I turn around I can't see the teachers either. Sometimes I hold my ears so I can't hear the game. I want everyone to leave me alone. Maybe my teachers can still see me. I don't want to see them. I don't want to see the game. I want the game to be over.

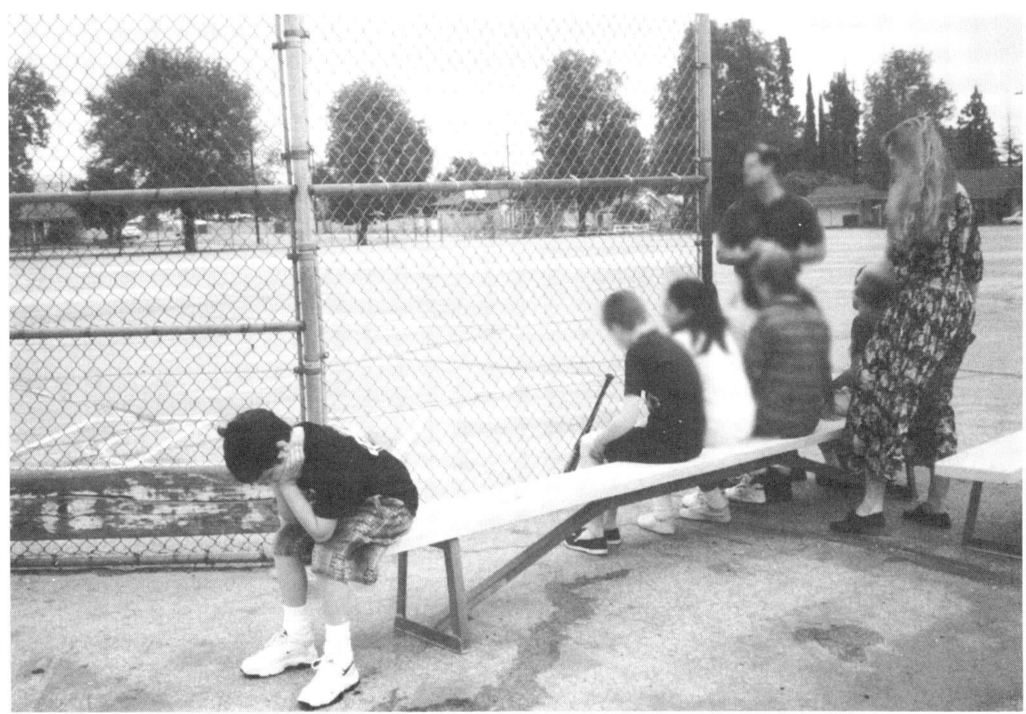

Sometimes I even lie down on the bench and pretend I am sleeping so everyone will leave me alone. This is not right. I am part of the team. The players are my friends. They need me to help them play better. I need to help them by trying my best to hit the ball and run to the bases. Maybe I can learn to play and help my team. Then maybe I can like to play baseball.

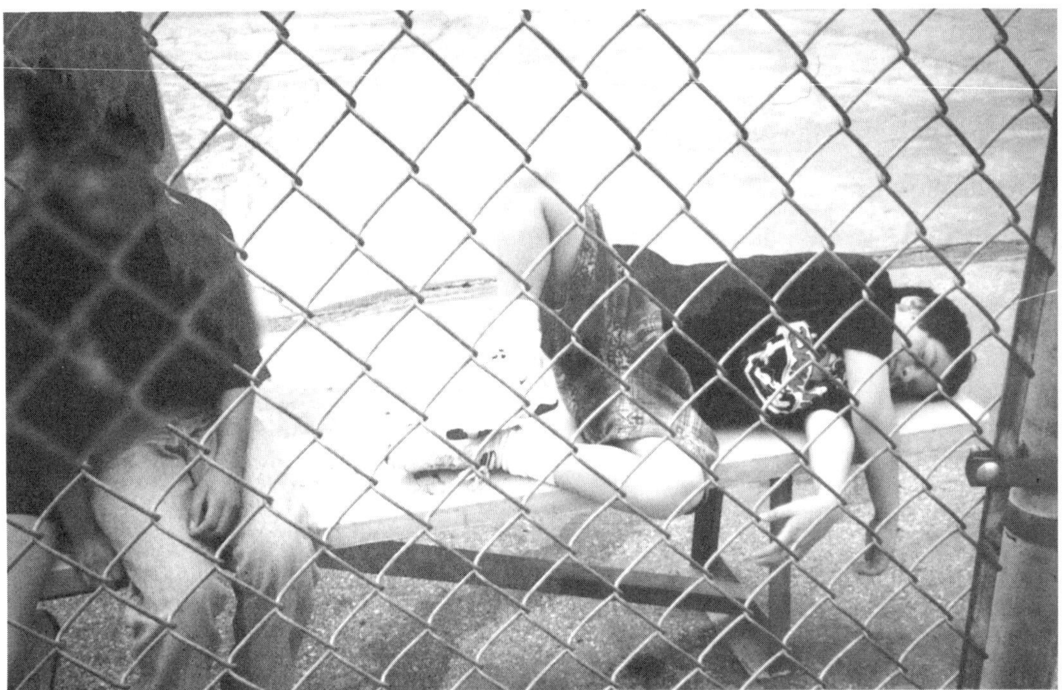

How can I learn about baseball? How can I learn to play baseball? Maybe I can ask my teachers to help me. Maybe I can ask my Dad to help me learn too. Maybe I can even ask my brother to teach me how to play baseball.

Learning about baseball may not be easy. But I am very smart. I think I can do it! I'm going to imagine a baseball game right now. I'm going to pretend I understand the rules. I'm going to pretend I already know how to play baseball.

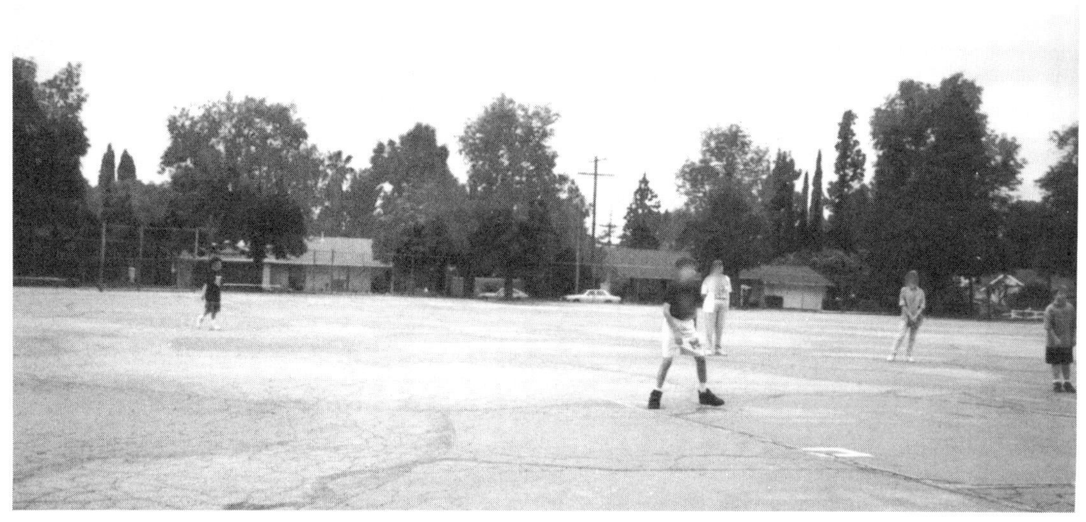

Chapter 2

Baseball games at school can be different from baseball games at the baseball stadium or on television. When we play baseball at school there are two teams. Our class is on one team and another class is on the other team. The two teams take turns. When our team is "up" we sit on the bench and wait for our turn to hit the ball. Everyone in our class gets a turn to hit the ball. When our team is up the other team is in the outfield. That means they try to catch the balls that we hit. They try to prevent us from running around all the bases. They want to keep us from making runs. They want to get us out.

When our team is sitting on the bench I try to watch each person on my team. When I watch what other people do I can learn about baseball. Watching is good. Watching is important. Every person on my team gets to try to hit the ball. They come up to home plate. They have a baseball bat in their hands. This is called being at bat.

When it is my turn, I get a baseball bat and walk up to home plate. I hold the bat just like the other kids do. The pitcher will pitch the ball to me and I try to hit it. I want to hit it very hard so it flies high up in the sky. I want it to fly very far. I want to hit it so hard that it flies to the end of the schoolyard. I want to hit it so hard and so far that while someone on the other team runs to get the ball I can run to first base. I need to put my foot on the base before I can run to the next base.

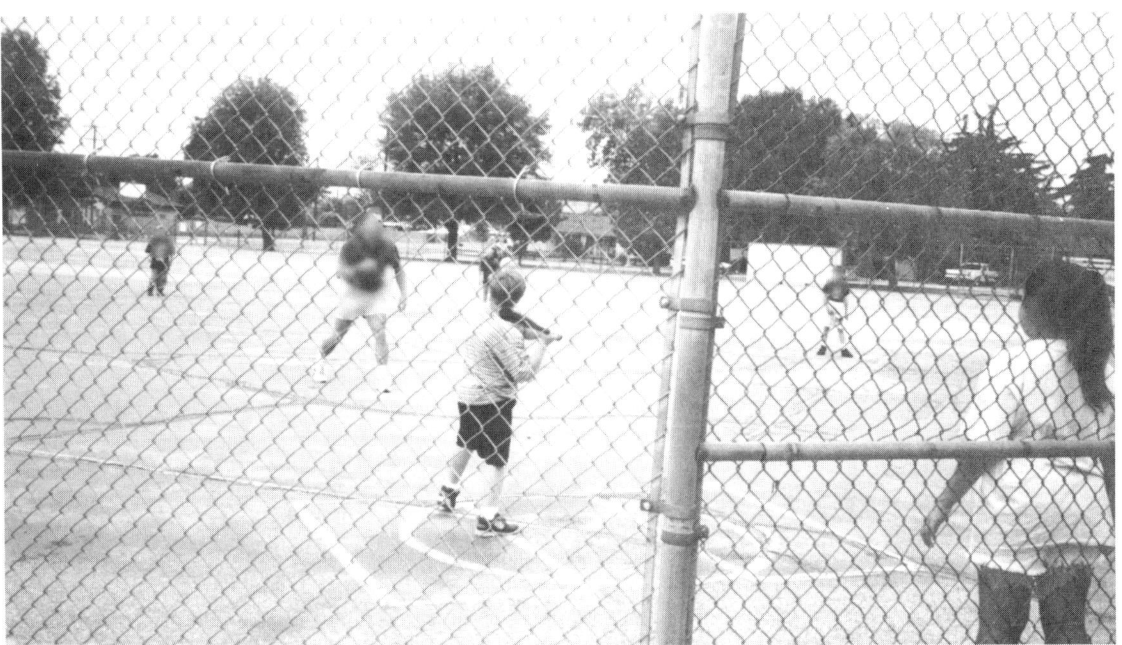

After I get to first base I need to look around. If the other team is still chasing the ball, then I may want to run to second base. I need to remember to touch each base as I run by it. I need to touch the base. Baseball players usually touch the base with their foot.

If players in the outfield are still chasing the ball I hit, I can even run to third base, and maybe even all the way to home plate. Wow! When this happens I have scored one run for our team.

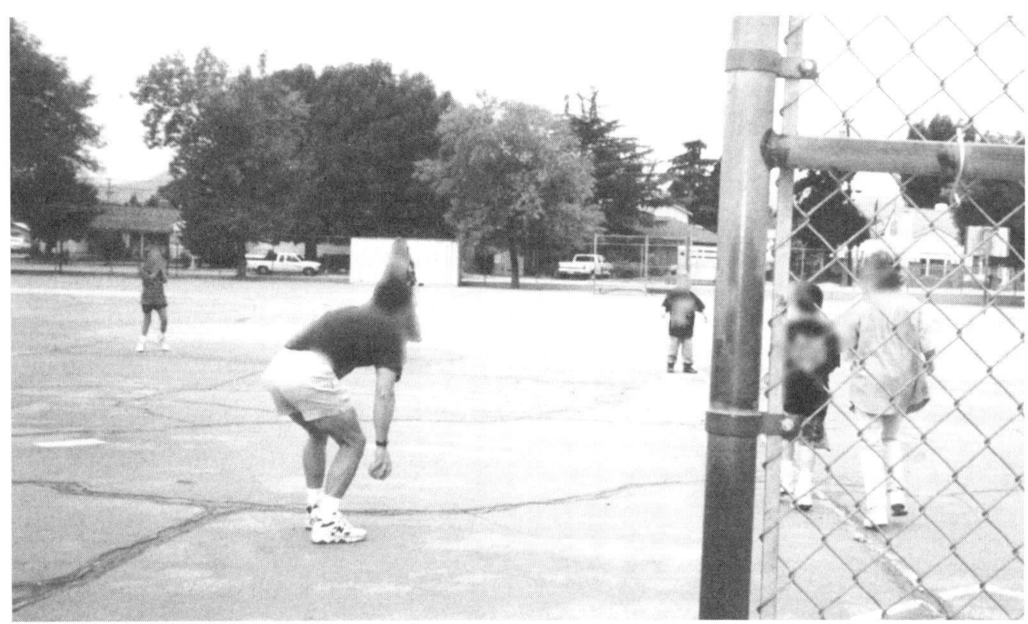

But, maybe I did not hit the ball very hard. Maybe I could only run to first base. If I only get to first base, then my teammates will each try to hit the ball to help me get to the other bases. In baseball, the whole team helps each other so the team can win. My teammates will try to help me get to other bases by hitting the ball as hard as they can. That is how we help each other. That is how we try to make runs. That is how we try to win the baseball game. At the end of the game, the team that has the most runs wins.

Chapter 3

Each member of a team is called a player. When we play baseball, each player is allowed to be at bat only one time each time our team is up. This is different from baseball games on television. This is different from baseball games at the stadium or in video games.

In the baseball games at school the pitcher will throw the ball to the player at bat three times. If the player does not hit the first ball that the pitcher throws, then the umpire, a special person who knows all the rules and makes decisions, may call out words like "strike one." If the player does not hit the second ball, the umpire may call out words like "strike two." If the player does not hit the third ball, the umpire may call out words like "strike three."

If this happens, the player has made an out and he sits back down on the bench. Now another player on our team comes up to the plate, takes a bat, and gets ready to try to hit the ball.

If I am standing on a base waiting to run and the next player at bat does not hit the ball after three pitches, I cannot go to the next base. I need to stay where I am. I need to wait for a player at bat to hit the ball before I can run toward the next base. In a baseball game on television or in a stadium the players can do other things, like steal a base. But we have different rules at school. We need to just stay on the same base until the batter hits the ball and starts running toward the first base.

After each player on our team has had a chance to hit the ball, our team changes places with the other team. Now we go into the outfield and the other team is up.

When our team goes into the outfield and the other team comes up to bat everything is different. Now it is our job to catch the balls that the other team tries to hit. Each player on our team tries to catch a ball that can be hit to him or her. If it is my job to be at first base, then another player on my team can be at second base or third base or shortstop or right field or center field or left field. We can all work together.

If I am the catcher, then another player on my team will take care of first base. We use special words to tell about staying in an area and guarding it. We say, "we play first base," "we play second base," "we play third base," "we play short stop," "we play right field," "we play center field," "we play left field," "we play catcher," "we play pitcher."

If I am the catcher, I catch each ball the batter does not hit. Then I throw the ball back to the pitcher so he can pitch it to the batter again.

If I play first base and the batter hits the ball, I try to catch the ball and touch the base with my foot, before the batter gets to it. If I can touch the base before the batter gets there, then the batter, who is now called a runner, is out. That means he has to go and sit back down on the bench. That means he will not be able to make a run. He will need to wait for each of the other members of his team to have a turn being at bat.

If I play second base, I try to catch the ball and touch the runner with it before he steps on second base. This is called tagging the runner. When a runner has been tagged before he touches the base, he is out. Then he will go back to his seat on the bench. He cannot make a run.

If I play third base, I try to catch the ball and touch the runner with it before he touches third base so that he will be out. Then he will go back to his seat on the bench. He cannot make a run.

If I play shortstop or right field or center field or left field and the ball is hit to me, then I try to catch the ball and throw it to a player who is guarding a base. I throw it toward the player as fast as I can so that he can tag the runner before that runner touches the base. If the runner touches the base before someone can tag him with the ball, then he is safe and can keep trying to finish going around all the bases until he makes a run.

A team makes a run when a player has gone safely from first base through second base, through third base and all the way to home plate without being tagged with the ball.

Baseball is what is called a team sport. This means that every person on the team works together. We work together so we can try and get more runs than the other team. The team that has the most runs at the end of the game wins the game.

Chapter 4

I would like to become a good baseball player. I will become a good baseball player if I look and listen and try my best when we play baseball at school.

I will become a better baseball player if I ask a question whenever I don't understand something that happens in a baseball game.

I will become a better baseball player if I practice with my Dad and my Mom and my brothers.

If I ask nicely, maybe my Dad will take me to the store and buy me a baseball bat and a baseball glove and a baseball and hat. Then we can practice at home together and have fun.

Maybe baseball really is fun, when you know how to play. I want to have fun; so, I'm going to learn how to play baseball.

The End

Not only is a good SF story worth its weight in gold, the pictures or photos accompanying the story tell a story as well. The few photographs in the baseball story tell a story all by themselves. They reveal a youngster who appears to be ill or tired or bored or sad. Yet the game goes on without him. He knows the other children in the photographs. They are his classmates and his teammates. They have significance to him.

Note that the story is mostly descriptive. It encourages him to do certain things and tells him why it is important to do these things. In this case, the story also addresses how I perceived he felt about the game. I could only do this because I felt I knew what he was feeling. Had I been wrong, he would not have responded as well as he did.

Within a few days I received a second telephone call. This call came from the classroom instructor. "We can't seem to prevent your son from going into another student's desk. We have repeatedly asked him not to do this, but our requests have thus far been ignored. He has also ventured into my desk a few times," said the instructor, a bit more concerned.

I assured her I would take care of the problem. Back to the school I went the following day, camera over my shoulder and pad and pencil in hand. I took photos of the desk he shared with a fellow student. I asked questions and got a better understanding of the problem. Within a few days the story was written. Like its predecessor, it worked well. He would no longer put his hands into his neighbor's desk nor his teacher's desk. He had begun to ask for permission in order to do so. In addition, when he was denied permission, he could restate the reasons why his request was rejected and said he would ask again at another time. Remember, you can always expand a story or change a story. A story that is fun and informative can make a world of difference to these wonderful individuals. We have included this SF story example below.

SF Story Example 2:

RESPECTING OTHER PEOPLE'S PROPERTY

Jill and I share a desk. I sit on one side of the desk and Jill sits on the other side of the desk. I have my chair and Jill has her chair. I keep my things inside my side of the desk and on top of the desk. Jill keeps her things inside her side of the desk and on top of the desk too. Jill's things belong to her. My things belong to me.

Sometimes I think Jill has something inside her desk that I might like to see and touch. But these things belong to Jill. They do not belong to me. I may not put my hands inside Jill's side of the desk. That is wrong. If I want to look at something inside her desk I need to look at Jill and ask her nicely. I need to say, "May I see something in your desk, Jill?" If she says yes, she may ask me what I want to see. Then she may decide to reach inside her desk. Only Jill can get things out of her desk. I may not. That is because the things inside Jill's desk belong to Jill.

If Jill does not want to share her things then she will say "No." And that is okay. I need to respect Jill's words. I may not get angry with Jill if she says no. Maybe she will share her things with me on another day. Sometimes I don't like to share my things and sometimes other people are not ready to share their things.

My teacher has her desk and her things. My teacher has a very big desk. She has many things on the top of her desk. She can open her desk drawers.

Sometimes I walk over to my teacher's desk. My teacher's desk is like Jill's desk. My teacher's desk belongs to my teacher. The things on the top of the desk belong to my teacher and the things inside of the desk belong to my teacher. I have my own desk and my own things.

I may not touch my teacher's desk. That would be wrong. I will try my best to stay away from my teacher's desk. I can be at my own desk. Then I will be proud of myself.

Each morning, when I come into the classroom, I can try very hard to remember to touch only the things that belong to me. Then my teacher will be happy. She will smile at me and say happy words to me. I am so proud of myself. I am wonderful. Hurrah for me!

Chapter XIII

The Social Album Model (SA)

The Social Album is really a variation of the SF Story model. You might even say the social album is an SF story. The social album can be used for individuals at all levels. However the Social Album is the model of choice for those individuals who, for any number of reasons, require fewer words, shorter, less complex sentences, using a larger type, and more photographs or drawings, etc., in order to better understand what we are attempting to convey.

Just as you and I never seem to tire of seeing old photo albums and reliving past experiences, so too the Social Album can provide a similar set of good feelings as well as vital information to the many individuals with special needs who might not be able to derive significant understanding of necessary information from, or be quite ready for, the SF story format.

In the case where a young individual is better suited to seeing photographs of themselves and others in various situations and places in order to convey vital information and understanding, the social album can be the ideal way to provide this information and understanding.

The social album contains as few words as is necessary to get vital information across. Since, however, there are fewer words, these words need to be as succinct and useful as possible. The words will need to pinpoint specific areas of concern providing understanding with few words and the greater use of other props.

Within the social album we can even use other items, such as pictures of special characters that the individual at risk finds comforting and familiar. Photos of everything from stop signs to cartoon characters can serve a purpose. Magazine pictures, concrete small items taped to a page, scents, all can enhance the experience.

I know someone with an eleven-year-old son who is not quite ready to read yet. His language skills are modest. Yet, it is apparent that hc has much to say. He knows and understands far more than his words would allow us to believe. His mother knows that his favorite character this year is Godzilla. When they are out and about she always carries a small notebook. At those moments when his behavior begins to break down she opens her bag and takes out the few sheets containing the pictures and words that are so comforting and reassuring to her son. Out comes Godzilla! Though this notebook does not provide him with new information about the world around him, it does enable his mother to continue her outing with him a bit longer.

For this child I have told her she can take Godzilla pictures and begin to weave a story or two for him relating to their upcoming journey for the day. In other words, she could use Godzilla to help her convey something of importance to him. For example, if her goal is to get him new shoes, she could put shoes on a picture of Godzilla. She could then place a photo of her son and pictures of new shoes next to that of Godzilla. She could write out a few simple words to convey to him that shoes are important. They are important to Godzilla and they are important for him. This day the three of them, herself, the photos of Godzilla and her son, are going to go on an outing to get him new shoes. It may sound silly, but it could help. For a visit to the dentist she could use Godzilla's teeth and a picture of the dentist and a toothbrush. In this way she could help prepare him for a visit to the dentist. Taking a picture or a group of pictures of someone or something the child likes and relating it to some future event can be more than helpful and disarming. It can give the individual knowledge as well as some control over future events. In this case upcoming knowledge of what to expect can give the child a sense of some control, something he may often seem to lack. He can anticipate and make himself ready for upcoming events. He has control over the unknown, which has now become known to him. Now his outing with his mother is something of a joint venture.

Social albums, however, are usually longer than the Godzilla model above and, in addition, they usually convey some understanding of a concept. Like the SF story, the social album seeks to explain some important concept or group of concepts. Defining and explaining friendship, how to be a friend and make a friend, can be accomplished through a social album just as it can be done through the SF story. A social album providing an understanding of the concept of stranger can be created as well. In fact, just about any information created in SF story form can be recreated in social album form. It is only a matter of design.

Below you will find an example of a social album. Note the fact that the album is not random. Instead, just as a quick-script or SF story, the social album is succinct, logical and sequential. It provides understanding in a way all its own. For those whose needs can best be served by the use of the social album, the results can be uplifting, positive and developmentally sound.

In the social album below note the use of large letters and small letters as well as the arrangement of the words and the spaces for photographs or other kinds of pictures. The entire story is created in such a way as to promote interest so that a story, such as this one, can be used repeatedly in order to enable understanding.

Social Album Example:

Using my

WORDS

Words can help me.
Words are important.
Words are like magic.
Words can tell people how I feel.
Words can tell people what I want.
Friends use their words.

When I want to play with the blue ball and my friend wants to play with the blue ball,
I need to use my words.

WORDS ARE SAFE!

[leave sufficient space between paragraphs and place a snapshot of the blue ball here]

Words can tell my friend what I want.

"I want to play with the blue ball," I can tell my friend.

My friend can use his words, too.

His words tell me what he wants.

Maybe he will say,

"I want to play with the ball, too."

Now it is my turn to talk.

Now it is my turn to use my words.

Maybe I can say, "Let's take turns."

Maybe I can say, "Let's share the ball."

Then we can both have fun.
Then we can both be happy.

But what if my friend says, "NO!"

What if my friend does not want to share?

What can I do?

[leave sufficient space between paragraphs and place a snapshot of the friend playing with the ball here]

I can use **MORE WORDS!**

What can I do if my friend
still will not share the ball?

Can I grab the ball? **No!**

I may not grab. Grabbing is not nice.

Grabbing is not being safe.

If I grab the ball, my friend may feel hurt.

If I grab the ball, my friend may not want to be my friend.

Can I hit my friend? **No!**

I may not hit. Hitting hurts.

Hitting is not being safe.

If I hit my friend, he will be hurt.

If I hit my friend, he may not want to be my friend.

Can I kick my friend? **No!**

I may not kick. Kicking hurts.

Kicking is not being safe.

If I kick my friend, he will be hurt.

If I kick my friend, he may not want to be friend.

Can I bite my friend? **No!**

I may not bite. Biting hurts.

Biting is not being safe.

If I bite my friend, he will be hurt.

If I bite my friend, he may not want to be my friend.

What can I do?

[leave sufficient space between paragraphs and place a snapshot of the child talking here]

I can use MORE WORDS.

I can use more words and more words and more words and more words and more words and more words and more words and more words.

I can use so many words that my friend may say YES!

Let's take turns!

Let's share!

[leave sufficient space between paragraphs and place a snapshot of a happy child here]

And all because of WORDS!

HURRAH FOR WORDS!

Chapter XIV

Social Interactive Adventures (SIA)

Remember back to when you were a youngster. Remember make-believe. Remember the rainy days and rainy-day playmates, the times you dressed up in Mom's and Dad's clothing, shoes and hats. Remember mud pies. Remember playing Superman, playing war, playing house and setting up those tea parties using miniature, plastic, toy tea cups. Remember the tiny toy cooking oven that actually allowed you to bake tiny, gritty cakes. Remember pretending you were Dad going to work or Mom teaching a lesson.

Do you remember the organizational spoofs you may have engaged in as you grew, the skits, the plays, the short, funny scenarios you put on, perhaps before a willing audience around a campfire on a warm summer night? What we did when we took part in these activities was to play out scenarios based on our previous exposure to situations. What we were doing was playing out various roles that would help in our social development. We had been exposed to the roles each parent played in our lives. We had watched Superman defend the weak and capture the bad guys. Remember make believe situations or real life ones and you are remembering some kind of learning situation.

For most of us, life is full of these special moments we played out, these "Social Interactive Adventures," or SIA's. What we may not have realized is how useful they would be to our social development.

Normally, each of us learns not only our own role in social interactions, but the roles of others by watching and mentally cataloging the scripts. We then know what role to play and how to play it, hence our social interactions are appropriate. For some individuals, however, these social interactive adventures are missing. There are few, if any. Until now, that is.

Recognizing the importance of these Social Interactive Adventures, or SIA's, we knew how essential a learning tool they would be within the SF framework. The Social Interactive Adventure could prove to be a cornerstone in the Social Facilitation process. We had recognized the importance of SIA's in social development and that their use would be beneficial and effective because SIA's would enable the individual at risk to begin to "experience," to feel and see and touch and be touched in a controlled manner within the framework of a particular social situation. So many of these individuals never played house or movie roles. So many of them had remained on the outside, perhaps never even looking inside a situation, never recognizing the experiential learning they were missing out on, never having engaged in the enjoyment.

Our goal in Social Facilitation was to help these special individuals to take part in these experiential forms of learning now. SIA's appear to be comfortable and fun. They are designed to be that way so that there will be less hesitancy or fear to use them.

More than fun, however, SIA's are instructive. With script in hand, these special individuals would no longer be on the outside, shut out, and shut off. The SIA process would gently help them, gently ease them in to a previously foreign, troubling or confusing situation. The social interactive adventure would plop them right down into some common social situation in life and allow them to play a specific social role. And not play that role just once, but over and over again, as many times as would be necessary, until it can be played with ease, comfort and security; and until any anxiety associated with taking part in it was reduced or extinguished.

Though it is possible to create a Social Interactive Adventure in monologue form (in which case the audience would become a non-interactive partner), the SIA is almost always set up between two or more individuals. Using focused scripts, the individuals in these skit-like scenarios practice social situations. Each person in an adventure has a role to play. Each person carries out that role using his or her script.

As the social adventure is repeatedly played out, roles may be switched. In this way each participant is given the opportunity to "feel and experience" what it is like to be in the other's place. The adventures can be used by all kinds of participants, children, adults, those at risk and those not at risk. It can often be helpful to have unimpaired peers of the individual at risk take part in the SIA process.

Through repeated and playful social interactions, the individual at risk can begin to let go of his need for isolation and withdrawal. Through the adventure process, it is hoped that he can begin to overcome anxiety and become more comfortable with the give and take that social interactions involve. And the more the individual begins to engage in this experiential process, the more, we believe, he can develop a kind of social awareness and social strength, so that he is able to learn to successfully engage and respond quickly and appropriately to social situations. See Chapter XVIII for sample SIA's based on everyday type of experiences.

PART II

Chapter XV

Quick Script Sample

Camp Schedule

Earlier in the manual we talked about a quick-script sample using a camp schedule and map. In that context we had put the schedule on a sheet of paper. You might remember that the back side of that paper had a map of the camp. We had put it in flyer form and had had it laminated. This is all possible. However, in reality, the "real story" did not allow time for the lamination process to take place. In the real story that morning two sheets of paper were used. The daily schedule was quickly typed and placed on one side of the sheet and an explanation of what the schedule means was placed on the other. Both sides were put in one clear plastic paper protector. Here is what was written:

[Side One]

A camp schedule tells me what will happen in a camp day.
A schedule can help me know what comes next.
Sometimes schedules change to make more fun.
On some days the schedule will stay the same.
Every day at camp is special.
Every day at camp can be fun.
I can take this schedule to camp with me.
I can put it on my wall next to my bed.
I can look at it every day and I can be happy.

[Side Two]

My Camp Schedule

Wake up time
Breakfast
Morning Services
Clean up
Fun activity
Lunch
Canteen
Rest Time
Kitah (class)
Swimming
More Fun Activities
Dinner
More Fun and fun and fun!
Good night!

Perhaps the most important use for the quick script pad is damage control. Its uses are endless. It is an on-the-spot method for allowing us to communicate vital information in order to help our special needs adults and children. It is a superb way to help us help them restore order to their lives and lower anxiety.

You stop at the supermarket to buy some milk and cereal. Bill, your eighteen-year-old son, has accompanied you. He loves Loop-D-Loop Cereal and you need another box. Bill pushes the shopping cart down the cereal aisle. He enjoys pushing the cart. Lo and behold, the supermarket is out of Loop-D-Loop Cereal. Not one box remains. Bill lets go of the cart and begins to pace. He utters some low growling sounds.

In the past, this situation might have posed a serious problem. But, all that has changed. You now have a tool in your purse to help you and Bill get through this potentially upsetting situation. You open your purse and grab your Quick Script pad and pen. The pad gives you confidence in your ability to get Bill to understand what has happened, why, and how it can be resolved.

Bill comes over and stands next to you as you write. Looking at the various choices to help you quickly determine Bill's emotional state you take your best guess and move on to the situation level. You acknowledge Bill's probable disappointment and possible confusion at finding the favorite cereal missing from the store shelf. Though Bill's ability to speak and respond in sentences is somewhat limited, he can read and is a good visual learner. You fill in the script pad sheet. He may respond as you write and he reads. Toward the end, you offer Bill a choice as to whether you should go on to another supermarket to find Loop-D-Loop Cereal or wait until tomorrow. You help Bill decide to take a chance and make the decision for him. Had your words been unacceptable to him, Bill would have let you know by word or emotional response. However, this decision was okay with him. Bill and Mom would return the following day to look again for Loop-D-Loop Cereal. All is well!

Quick Script Pad

Identify Emotion(s): sad frustrated confused mad disappointed angry bored hurt other ________

Situation: Insert name/pronoun + emotion(s) + problem:

Bill feel(s) ***disappointed & confused***

because: ***The Loop-D-Loop Cereal is not here on the shelf where we usually find it. Bill loves Loop-D-Loop Cereal.***

Getting Help (information): ***Let's talk to the store manager and find out what has happened to the cereal. The manager says that many people like to buy and eat Loop-D-Loop Cereal. The manager says he will have lots of Loop-d-Loop Cereal tomorrow at 2:00 p.m.***

List Options/Choices: ***We can come back tomorrow after 2:00 p.m. and buy Loop-D-Loop Cereal at this supermarket or we can go to another supermarket right now and buy Loop-D-Loop Cereal. What would you like to do? Would you like to come back tomorrow? Good choice, Bill!***

Action Taken: ***Bill & Mom will come back at 2:00 p.m. tomorrow and buy Loop-D-Loop Cereal. Then Bill can go home and eat it.***

Concluding Feelings: ***Bill can be happy now because he knows that tomorrow his Loop-D-Loop Cereal will be here and we will buy it.***

Upon entering a shopping mall, a mother turns to her two sons with special needs and promises to buy them each a cupcake. The two boys are delighted. Soon they find themselves in a muffin shop. The mother purchases two chocolate chip muffins for the boys. "Here are your chocolate chip muffins, boys" she says. No sooner does she hand the first boy his muffin, which he takes in his hands and proceeds to eat, than the second boy flings himself on the floor, arms and legs flailing about along with assorted shrill screams. The mother can't understand what the problem could be. She tries and tries to coax him to quiet down and tell her the problem. It seems that the harder she tries, the more upset the youngster becomes. She looks at the second muffin. It looks scrumptious. She is totally bewildered until she thinks a minute more. All was well until the word muffin appeared, she thought.

Though she knows that a quick script usually works best before a full-blown tantrum is underway, she reaches into her purse to get out her pad. She writes:

Quick Script Pad

Identify Emotion(s): sad <u>frustrated</u> confused mad

disappointed <u>angry</u> bored hurt other ________________

Situation: Insert name/pronoun + emotion(s) + problem:

I see that you ________ feel(s) ***frustrated and angry***

because: ***you are lying on the floor.***

Getting Help (information): ***A muffin is a cupcake.***

A muffin is a delicious kind of cupcake. And a chocolate chip muffin cupcake is the best one of all.

List Options/Choices: ***This is the cupcake I promised you.***

Action Taken: ***Please come and eat your cupcake.***

Concluding Feelings: ***It is fun to eat muffins together.***

This muffin cupcake tastes yummy! We can be happy when we eat muffins.

This quick script did not need to be very long. Because the child had already resorted to a full-blown temper tantrum he could not even hear his mother tell him that a muffin was a kind of cupcake. On the backside of the script sheet she had also written in big letters, "A MUFFIN IS A CUPCAKE." That got his attention. The front side provided the details. Once the child understood that the muffin was, indeed, the cupcake he had been promised, his world was restored to order. He got right up from the floor and sat down at the table to eat, as if nothing had happened.

Chapter XVI

Sample SF Story

A mother came to me with a problem. Her son kept putting things up his nose and in his ears. She had already taken him to the doctor on more than one occasion to remove the objects from each. She was, of course, quite concerned. This is what we came up with to help solve the problem.

When reading through the story please note that several important, relevant questions had been asked. One important question surrounded the child's possible fear of bugs and germs. There were none. In addition, the question was asked pertaining to fears and possible obsessions to what might be written. Telling the mother what was planned we developed the following:

My Nose and My Ears

It is important to take good care of my body. Taking care of my body can help me stay healthy. If I don't take good care of my body I may get sick or hurt. I don't want to be sick. I don't like to get hurt.

Putting things in my ears can hurt me. It is bad for my ears. I remember in *Star Trek 2* when Kahn put the ugly bug into the man's ears. His ears hurt. He cried.

Ears are delicate. Putting things in my ears may make me cry just like the man in *Star Trek 2*. This is because things that I put into my ears may have little germs on them. I can't see the germs. Germs can hurt me. Germs may hurt my ears. Germs can infect my ears. Then I would have an ear infection. Ear infections can hurt more than headaches. I don't want germs in my ears. I don't want an ear infection. I don't want to cry. So, I will not put things in my ears. Then they can be healthy. Then they can hear their very best.

Putting things into my nose is bad for me, too. My nose is very important. I smell through my nose. I breathe air that goes into my lungs through my nose. This air feeds my whole body. When air enters my nose it goes past little villi. The little villi clean the air. They take dirt and dust out of the air so that it can't go into my lungs. If I put my finger or a bead or something else inside my nose I stop the air from coming into my nose. Then the villi cannot do their job. The villi may even get hurt. If the villi are hurt the air will not be cleaned before it enters my lungs. If something is in my nose it could prevent air from going into my lungs. This is not good.

If I put something into my nose it could even go up into my brain. It could even get stuck. Then I might have to go to the hospital so the doctor can take it out. This is not good.

Putting my finger into my nose looks awful. If I put my finger there, people may look at me and frown. People know that fingers and other things do not belong inside a nose. I don't want people to frown at me. That might make me sad.

I want to be happy. I want people to say nice things to me. I want people to smile at me.

If something is in my nose I need to ask for a tissue or a handkerchief to take it out. Then I can blow my nose. Blowing my nose to clean it is good. Using a tissue or a handkerchief to blow my nose is the right thing to do.

I will try to remember not to put things into my ears and my nose, no matter what! I am wonderful! Hurrah for me!

Chapter XVII

Sample Social Album

<u>STRANGERS</u>

A STRANGER IS SOMEONE I DON'T KNOW!

A stranger can be big.

A stranger can be small.

A stranger can be old.

A stranger can be young.

A stranger can be a man.

A stranger can be a lady.

People I do not know are strangers.
Strangers may not be safe.
Strangers can be scary.

Stranger sounds like
Danger.

Stranger can mean Danger.

Danger means I may get hurt.

Danger means I am not safe.

I am not safe if I am with a stranger.

I may be in danger if I am with a stranger.

A stranger may say my name.

But I don't know the stranger's name.

So I may not talk to a stranger.

No matter what?

No matter what!

I may not walk with a stranger.

Because **stranger** can mean **danger.**

I may not ride in a car with a stranger.

Because **stranger** can mean **danger.**

I may not take things to eat from a stranger.

Because **stranger** can mean **danger.**

I may not take toys from a stranger.

Because **stranger** can mean **danger.**

Strangers may not touch me.

And I may not touch strangers.

Even if they ask me to touch them.

No matter what?
No matter what!

Are strangers bad?
Sometimes strangers are bad.

Can strangers be good?
Sometimes strangers can be good.

But I am little.

I don’t know if a stranger is good.
I don’t know if a stranger is bad.

So I may not talk or walk or ride
or take food or toys from a stranger.

No matter what?
No matter what!

[leave sufficient space between paragraphs and place a snapshot of unfamiliar people here]

Are these people strangers? Yes!

I do not know these people.

People I do not know are strangers.
These people are strangers.

May I talk to these people?

No! I may not talk to these people.

I might not be safe.

May I go with these people?

No! I may not go with these people.

I might not be safe.

Should these people touch me?

No! These people should not touch me.

I might not be safe.

May I touch these people?

No! I may not touch these people.

May I hug these people?

No! I may not hug these people.

I might not be safe.

No matter what?

No matter what!

[leave sufficient space between paragraphs and place a snapshot of an unfamiliar individual here]

Is this person a stranger?

Yes! I do not know this person.

Someone I do not know is a stranger.
This person is a stranger.

What should I do if a stranger talks to me?

I need to run and tell someone I know.
Like my Mommy or Daddy or Grandma or Grandpa.
I need to use my words to tell about strangers.

Because words can help to keep me safe.

What should I do if a stranger touches me?

If a stranger touches me I need to run and tell someone I know.
I need to use my words to keep me safe.
No matter what?

Yes! No matter what!

My words can help to keep me safe.

My words are wonderful!

What should I do if a stranger tries to give me food or a toy?

May I take the food? May I take the toy?

No! No! No!

I need to run and tell someone I know.
What can I say? What can I do?
I can use my best words to tell about the stranger. Then I can be safe.

I may not take the food.
I may not take the toy.
No matter what?

No matter what!

Can animals be strangers, too?

Yes!

Animals I do not know are strangers.

If I do not know a cat or a dog they are strangers.

May I pet a dog that I do not know?
No! A strange dog could bite me.
That would hurt. Ouch!
I might be very sad.
I might cry.
I might even have to go to the doctor.

May I pet a cat I do not know?
No! A strange cat could scratch me.

That would hurt. Ouch!

I might be very sad.

I might cry.

I might even have to go to the doctor.

[leave sufficient space between paragraphs and place a snapshot of an unfamiliar dog here]

Is this dog a stranger?

Yes! I do not know this dog.

If I touch this dog he might bite me.

This dog is a stranger.

I need to be safe.

So I may not touch this dog.

[leave sufficient space between paragraphs and place a snapshot of an unfamiliar cat here]

Is this cat a stranger?

Yes! I do not know this cat.

If I touch this cat it could scratch me.

I need to be safe.

So I may not touch this cat.

[leave sufficient space between paragraphs and place a snapshot of familiar children here]

Are these children strangers?

No! These children are not strangers.

I know these children.

These children are not strangers.

These children are my friends.

May I talk to these children? Yes!

I may talk to these children because I know them.

I know their names.

And they know my name, too.

We play together.

We eat together.

We share.

[leave sufficient space between paragraphs and place a snapshot of Mother here]

Is Mommy a stranger?

No! Mommy is not a stranger.

I know Mommy.

I am safe with Mommy.

I feel good when I am with Mommy.

Mommy loves me and I love Mommy.

[leave sufficient space between paragraphs and place a snapshot of Father here]

Is Daddy a stranger?

No! Daddy is not a stranger.

I know Daddy.

I am safe with Daddy.

I feel good when I am with Daddy.

Daddy loves me and I love Daddy.

Being safe is very important.

I feel safe when I am with big people that I know.

I feel safe when I am with small people that I know.

I feel safe when I am with old people that I know.

I am safe when I am with young people that I know.

I am safe when I am with people that I know.

Being safe feels good.

[leave sufficient space between paragraphs and place a snapshot of the child with familiar people here]

I am terrific!

I don't walk with a stranger.

I don't talk to a stranger.

I don't take food from a stranger.

I don't take toys from a stranger.

I am very safe.

No matter what!

Chapter XVIII

Social Interactive Adventure Samples

A social interactive adventure can focus on any topic you choose. It can be at any level you choose, from the simplest to the most complex. The goal of the adventure is to create an interactive experience with the participants responding as they might in the given situation. The script created can be very positive and celebratory. It can be perplexing. It can unearth a potentially unpleasant dilemma and attempt to resolve it.

The goal here is to create a kind of interactive looping. By socially interactive looping we mean that the participants move the conversation forward as they complete each thought (closure), yet link the completed social transaction to another thought, back and forth, back and forth, progressing forward. What do we mean? Do you remember a toy called a "Slinky," a kind of metal coil with both a front end and a back end? You could take this toy and place it on top of a stairwell and begin its downward descent. First one part of the toy would descend to the next lower stair and then the back end of the toy would be pulled along to that next lowest stair. Then the process would repeat itself until it had reached the bottom of the stairwell, thus ending the descent and the toy's use. Interactive looping in the SIA serves the same purpose. One person says or does something and the next person responds. There may be give and take as to who proceeds next, but the process is still the same, stimulus and response, stimulus and response; each stimulus-response segment representing a kind of beginning-end, beginning-end. And yet, like the toy Slinky going down stair after stair, so too, these stimulus-response sequences are connected and continue to loop themselves forward until the script comes to an end.

We are including three sample SIA's in this manual. The ones we have chosen are targeted for children through ages fourteen or fifteen. Obviously, the ones we've selected can be used for other ages as well. In reality, there are literally hundreds of these SIA's that can and will be written. Because birthdays are usually both positive and special moments in the lives of so many of us, we decided that it would be appropriate to put a birthday SIA first.

Scene: *It's a special day at school. It's one youngster's birthday. His mom has just brought in cupcakes and ice cream for the whole class. Everyone is excited.*

Child #1: I didn't know today was your birthday. Happy birthday.

Child #2: Thanks.

Child #1: Those cupcakes look great. Are they for everyone?

Child #2: Yes. There's ice cream, too.

Child #1: What flavor?

Child #2: Vanilla.

Child #1: I kind of like chocolate better.

Child #2: I used to eat chocolate. My mom said some kids can't eat chocolate.

Child #1: What's inside the cupcakes?

Child #2: They're vanilla on the inside and the outside. I put the sprinkles on top.

Child #1: Your mom's nice. My mom never sends cupcakes and ice cream to school on my birthday.

Child #2: When's your birthday?

Child #1: Next month.

Child #2: Maybe you could ask your mom to bring cupcakes like my mom did.

Child #1: Maybe I will. My mom's a good baker.

Child #2: Do you like vanilla cupcakes?

Child #1: Yeah. But I still like chocolate cupcakes better.

Child #2: Me too. But my mom says I can't eat chocolate anymore. Makes me sick.

Child #1: What about lemon? Can you eat lemon cupcakes?

Child #2: I guess so. I think so.

Child #1: Sometimes we have this lemon cake at home. It's great.

Child #2: Maybe I could come over to your house for lemon cake.

Child #1: Yeah. I'll ask my mom if you can come over the next time she makes it. Anyway, happy birthday. I'm glad we're friends.

Child #2: Me too!

The second SIA takes place in a different setting and can be most helpful.

Scene: *Local family restaurant. It's lunchtime. It's noisy. A mother and her children have just come into the restaurant.*

Waitress: *(looking at family)* Would you like to sit by the window?

Mother: *(looking at sons)* Do you want to sit by the window, boys?

Son #1: I do.

Son #2: Me too.

Mother: *(looking at the waitress)* The window will be fine.

(As they arrive at the table one son speaks up)

Son #1: It's too noisy in here. I don't like noise.

Son #2: It's not that noisy. C'mon. Don't complain.

Son #1: You don't care about noise like I do. All the people talking bugs me.

Son #2: Get used to it. Lots of places are noisy. You are the one who wanted to eat here. Hold your ears if the noise is so bad.

Son #1: *(doesn't like the noise but wants to stay. Turns toward his Mother)* All this noise hurts my ears.

Waitress: *(anxious to help)* There is another table on the other side of the restaurant. It is much quieter there.

Mother: *(looking at her sons)* Would you like to go to the other side of the restaurant?

Son #1: Yes.

Son #2: *(Shrugs shoulders)* I don't care.

(They are all seated and receive menus)

Mother: What do you want to eat, kids?

Son #1: I don't know.

Son #2: A hamburger, French fries and a lemon-lime soda.

Son #1: *(a moment later)* Chicken nuggets and onion rings and a cola.

Mother: I think I'll have a salad.

(The waitress writes down the order. A few minutes pass.)

Son #1: How come it takes so long for the food to come?

Son #2: There you go again. Complaining as usual.

Son #1: No I don't. I just don't like to wait so long.

Mother: It takes the cook a while to make the food we order. And there are other people who have ordered food. The cook has to make everyone's food.

Son #1: For the whole restaurant? It's going to take too long. We're going to miss the movie. I don't want to be late. We shouldn't have come here.

Mother: We have plenty of time, son. Look at your wristwatch. Everything is just fine. Lunch will be here soon. We're going to have a lovely day.

The third SIA relates to a sharing day at school.

Scene: *One youngster has brought her pet turtle to class. The whole class is curious. Two friends are standing next to her. They are anxious to touch the turtle. She becomes worried about the safety of her pet.*

Student #1: *(looking at a second student)* Stop grabbing at my turtle. You'll hurt him.

Student #2: I'm not grabbing. I'm looking.

Student #3: Can I hold the turtle?

Student #1: This is my share day and I am the only one who can hold my turtle.

Student #3: That's not fair. You're supposed to share on your share day.

Student #2: Yeah. If you won't share your turtle we won't be your friends.

Student #3: C'mon. We won't hurt him. We'll be careful.

Student #2: Yeah. We'll be really careful.

Student #1: Well, okay, but remember you promised.

(hold a piece of paper with the word turtle printed on it or hold a picture of a turtle)

Student #3: *(giggles)* His feet are tickling me.

Student #2: Let me hold him.

Student #1: *(takes the turtle from one student and hands him to the second one. He begins to giggle too)*

Student #2: It tickles. Can I hold him for a while?

Student #1: For one more minute. Then I need to put him back in his box. He's getting tired.

Student #2: *(holds him for one more minute)* How do you know he's getting tired? Maybe he likes me to hold him.

Student #1: I have to put him away. You had your turn.

Student #2: *(gives back turtle to Student #1)* He's great. I think I'll ask my aunt to get me a turtle. She works in a pet store. They have turtles there. They have other animals too, even fish.

Student #3: I don't like fish. They're boring. I like birds.

Student #1: What kinds of animals are at your aunt's store?

Student #2: All kinds of puppies and birds and snakes.

Student #3: I don't like snakes. They're scary.

Student #2: No they're not. They're neat. They're kind of soft and slippery.

Student #1: Do you think snakes eat turtles?

Student #2: Maybe big snakes can.

Student #3: I don't think so. They probably eat birds though.

Student #1: Can you take us to your aunt's pet store the next time you go?

Student #3: Yeah. Can you?

Student #2: Maybe. I'll call my aunt when I get home from school. If she says we can come, I'll tell you at school tomorrow.

BIBLIOGRAPHY

Adams, Janice I. *Autism – P.D.D.: More Creative Ideas*. Ontario: Adams Publications, 1997.

Aichelburg, Peter C. and Roman U. Sexl. *Albert Einstein: His Influence on Physics, Philosophy and Politics*. Braunschweig/Wiesbaden: Friedr Vieweg and Sohn, 1979.

Angoff, Charles. *Science and the Human Imagination: Albert Einstein*. New York: Associated University Press, 1978.

Attwood, Tony. *ASPERGER'S SYNDROME: A Guide for Parents and Professionals*. London: Jessica Kingsley Publishers, 1998.

Barron, Judy and Sean Barron. *There's A Boy In Here*. New York: Simon & Schuster, 1992.

Beck, Anna, and Peter Havas. *The Collected Papers of Albert Einstein, The Early Years: 1879-1902*. Vol. 1. Princeton: Princeton University Press, 1987.

Beck, Anna, and Peter Havas. *The Collected Papers of Albert Einstein, The Swiss Years: Writings, 1900-1909*. Vol. 2. Princeton: Princeton University Press, 1989.

Bernstein, Jeremy. *Einstein* New York: The Viking Press, 1973.

Clark, Ronald W. *EINSTEIN: The Life And Times*. New York: Avon Books, 1984.

Copeland, Lewis. *The World's Greatest Speeches*. New York: Dover Publications, 1958.

De Broglie, Louis. *Einstein*. New York: Peebles Press, 1979.

Damasio, Antonio R. *Descartes' Error*. New York: Avon Books, 1994.

Dukas, Helen, and Banesh Hoffmann. *Albert Einstein: The Human Side*. Princeton: Princeton University Press, 1979.

Einstein, Albert. *Out Of My Later Years*. New York: Philosophical Library, 1950.

EINSTEIN, A Portrait. California: Pomegranate Books, 1984.

Einstein, Albert. *Letters to Slovine*. New York: Philosophical Library, 1982.

Frank, Philipp. *EINSTEIN, His Life and Times*. New York: Da Capo Press, 1947.

Gillingham, Gail. *Autism, Handle with Care!* Arlington: Future Horizons.

Goleman, Daniel. *Emotional Intelligence*. New York: Bantam Books, 1994.

Gray, Carol, ed. *The New Social Story Book*. Arlington: Future Horizons, 1994.

Hermanns, William. *Einstein and the Poet: In Search of the Cosmic Man*. Brookline Village: Branden Press, 1983.

Highfield, Roger, and Paul Carter. *Private Lives of ALBERT EINSTEIN*. New York: St. Martin's Press, 1993.

Hoffman, Banesh, and Helen Dukas. *Albert Einstein Creator and Rebel*. New York: The Viking Press, 1972.

Holton, Gerald, and Yehuda Elkana. *Albert Einstein: Historical and Cultural Perspectives*. Princeton: Princeton University Press, 1982.

Infeld, Leopold. *Albert Einstein: His Work and Its Influence On Our World*. New York: Charles Scribner & Sons, 1950.

Kelly, Kate and Peggy Ramundo. *You Mean I'm Not Lazy, Stupid Or Crazy?!* New York: Scribner, 1993.

Lanczos, Cornelius. *Albert Einstein and the Cosmic World Order*. New York: Interscience, 1965.

Michelmore, Peter. *EINSTEIN, Profile of the Man*. New York: Dodd, Mead & Company, 1962.

Miller, Susan Martins. *Reading Too Soon*. Elmhurst: Center For Speech and Language Disorders, 1993.

O'Neill, Jasmine Lee. *Through the Eyes of Aliens: A Book About Autistic People*. London: Jessica Kingsley Publishers, 1999.

Pais, Abraham. *Subtle is the Lord: The Science and the Life of Albert Einstein*. New York: Oxford University Press, 1982.

Pais, Abraham. *Einstein lived here*. New York: Oxford University Press, 1994.

Pinker, Steven. *The Language Instinct: How the Mind Creates Language*. New York: William Morrow and Company, 1994.

Pyenson, Lewis. *THE YOUNG EINSTEIN: The Advent of Relativity*. Bristol and London: Adam Hilger Ltd., 1985.

Ratey, John J. M.D. and Catherine Johnson Ph.D. *Shadow Syndromes* New York: Pantheon Books, 1995.

Sayen, Jamie. *Einstein In America*. New York: Crown Publishers, 1985.
Schilipp, Paul Arthur. *ALBERT EINSTEIN: Philosopher-Scientist*. Volume 1. London: Cambridge University Press, 1969.
Sosin, David & Myra Sosin. *Professional's Guide: Attention Deficit Disorder*. Westminster: Teacher Created Materials, 1996.
Stachel, John. *The Collected Papers of Albert Einstein, The Swiss Years: Writings, 1900-1909*. Vol. 2. Princeton: Princeton University Press, 1989.
Sugimoto, Kenji. *ALBERT EINSTEIN: A Photographic Biography*. New York: Schocken Books, 1989.
Vallentin, Antonina. *Einstein, A Biography*. London: Weidenfeld and Nicolson, 1984.
Williams, Donna. *An Inside-Out Approach*. London: Jessica Kingsley Publishers, 1996.
Williams, Donna. *SOMEBODY SOMEWHERE: Breaking Free from the World of Autism*. New York: Times Books, 1994.
Yellen, Andrew G. Ph.D. *The Art of Perfect Parenting and Other Absurd Ideas*. Northridge: Yellen & Associates, Northridge, 1993.

"After All, Einstein Is A Human Being," *Literary Digest* April 13, 1929:38-40.
"Baffled Sage," *Time* May 27, 1949:44.
"Einstein Fiddles," *Time* February 3, 1941:45.
"Einstein's Autobiography," *Newsweek* December, 1949:53.
"Einstein, The Man Behind The Genius," *Reader's Digest* August, 1972:23-30.
"Genius At Home," *Time* July 24, 1944:64-66.
Hoffman, Banesh, "Einstein, the genius who couldn't get a job," *Science Digest* February, 1973:32-37.
Hoffman, Banesh, "Unforgettable Albert Einstein," *Reader's Digest,* January, 1968:107-112.
"Is The Einstein Theory A Crazy Vagary?" *The Literary Digest* June 2, 1923:29-30.
Joralemon, Dorothy R. "When Einstein Sat for My Mother," *50 PLUS* June, 1982:22-25.
Marsh, Jeffrey; "Images of Einstein," *Commentary* December, 1972:65-70.
Overbye, Dennis. "Einstein In Love," *Time* April 30, 1990:108.
Schwartz, Daniel. "Einstein's Theory of Living," *Science Digest* March 12, 1944:55-59.
Snow, C.P. "Two Aspects of Science's Giant," *Life* August 20, 1971:14.
Stachel, John. "Einstein and Ether Drift Experiments," *Physics Today* May, 1987:45-47.
Viereck, George Sylvester. "What Life Means to Einstein," *The Saturday Evening Post* October 26, 1929:17, 110, 113-115.
Wheeler, John Archibald. "The Outsider," *Newsweek* March 12, 1979:67.
Walker, Evan Harris. "Mileva Maric's Relativistic Role," *Physics Today* February, 1991:122-124.

About the Authors

Illana Katz

Illana Katz is an award-winning author, lecturer, researcher, and Social Facilitation Consultant with Yellen & Associates. She is the recipient of the Authors and Celebrities "Award of Excellence" and the "Irwin Award" from Book Publicists of Southern California. She been consistently recognized by *Who's Who* in the West, in America and in the World. She has appeared on the *Today Show* as well as numerous other television and radio programs as an expert dealing with behavioral issues surrounding autism and Asperger's Syndrome. She has lectured nationwide and has been invited to speak in England and Europe. She has been featured in magazine and newspaper articles, and is a free-lance writer for the *Heritage* and the *Los Angeles Times*. Illana Katz is married and is the mother of four children, one of whom has autism.

Andrew G. Yellen, Ph.D.

Andrew Yellen has been a Clinical and Sports Psychologist for 16 years, with a practice in Northridge, California. Dr. Yellen has lectured nationally and internationally on behavioral management, parenting, Attention Deficit Disorder, and Tourette Syndrome. He has led seminars for hospital staffs and insurance corporations, and has worked closely with organizations designing crisis and substance abuse intervention models.

Among other professional affiliations, Dr. Yellen is a Fellow and Diplomate of the Prescribing Psychologists' Register and the American Board of Medical Psychotherapists. He is a member of the California, Los Angeles County, and San Fernando Valley Psychological Associations. Additionally, Dr. Yellen is an Irlen Diagnostician, identifying and treating Irlen Scotopic Sensitivity Syndrome. He has authored *The Art of Perfect Parenting and Other Absurd Ideas*, and together with Heidi Yellen, he co-authored *Understanding the Learning Disabled Athlete*. He has been interviewed on radio and television numerous times as a recognized expert on psychological issues.

Dr. Yellen began his professional career as an educator, and holds Standard Teaching, Community college, and Administrative Credentials.

Ordering Information

A variety of Social Facilitation materials is available for purchase. To order materials or a price list on-line, visit *www.socialfacilitation.com;* or write to: **Yellen & Associates, 11260 Wilbur Avenue, Suite 303, Northridge, CA 91326** or call Yellen & Associates at **(818) 360-3078, ext. 102.**

Types of literature available include:

- Quick Script Pads for you to fill in as needed
- Schedule Pads to make your daily travels together easier
- Social Facilitation (SF) Stories for various common situations
- SIA's (Social Interactive Adventures) for everyday life events
- Social Albums (add your own photos)
- Customized SF Stories, Social Albums, and SIA's--call (818) 360-3078 ext. 102 for prices.